LYME DISEASE COOKBOOK

5 Manuscripts in 1 – 240+ Recipes designed to manage Lyme Disease

TABLE OF CONTENTS

Introduction

Lyme Disease recipes for personal enjoyment but also for family enjoyment. You will love them for sure for how easy it is to prepare them.

BREAKFAST

CHOCOLATE COCONUT OATS

Serves: **4**

Prep Time: **10**   Minutes

Cook Time: **10**   Minutes

Total Time: **20**   Minutes

INGREDIENTS

- 1 cup oats
- 2 tablespoons chia seeds
- 2 tablespoons maple syrup
- 1 vanilla extract
- 1 tablespoon cocoa powder
- 1 cup water
- 2/3 cup coconut milk
- 2 tablespoons water

DIRECTIONS

1. In a bowl mix oat with water and place it in the fridge overnight
2. In the morning add chia seeds and coconut milk
3. Transfer mixture to a skillet and cook for 5 minutes

4. Remove and move into serving bowl and add vanilla extract, cacao powder and maple syrup

5. Serve when ready

QUINOA MUESLY WITH COCONUT MILK

Serves: **4**

Prep Time: **10**   Minutes

Cook Time: **10**   Minutes

Total Time: **20**   Minutes

INGREDIENTS

- 1 cup Quinoa
- ½ cup coconut milk yogurt
- 1 pinch ground cinnamon
- 1 cup Grain Free Muesli

DIRECTIONS

1. Cook the quinoa according to the indications, nd set aside

2. Drizzle the quinoa with coconut milk yogurt and top with grain free muesli, add cinnamon and serve

Serves: **4**

Prep Time: **10**   Minutes

Cook Time: **30**   Minutes

Total Time: **40**   Minutes

INGREDIENTS

- 3 sweet potatoes
- 8 tablespoons almond milk
- 1 tablespoon mint leaves
- 1 tablespoon lemon zest
- 1 tablespoon coconut oil
- 1 pinch salt
- 1 pinch ground cinnamon
- 3 tablespoons vanilla cereal

DIRECTIONS

1. Preheat oven to 350 F and line a baking sheet with parchment paper
2. Place the sweet potatoes on the baking sheet
3. Rub the sweet potato with coconut oil and sprinkle salt and pepper
4. Roast for 30 minutes

5. Remove the sweet potatoes from the oven and cut into small pieces

6. Top with coconut oil, lemon zest and cereal mixture

BANANA SPLIT

Serves: *2*

Prep Time: *10*   Minutes

Cook Time: *10*   Minutes

Total Time: *20*   Minutes

INGREDIENTS

- 2 bananas
- 1 cup strawberries
- 1 cup blackberries
- 1 cup chopped pineapple
- 1 cup coconut milk
- 1 tablespoon whole grain granola
- ¼ ounce roasted coconut chips

DIRECTIONS

1. Slice the bananas and place them into a bowl

2. Divide the strawberries, blackberries and pineapple and place it in the bottom of the bowl
3. Top with yogurt and divide the granola and coconut chips between the bananas

CHAI-SPICED PEAR OATMEAL

Serves: **2**

Prep Time: **10** Minutes

Cook Time: **30** Minutes

Total Time: **40** Minutes

INGREDIENTS

- 1 cup oats
- ½ tsp ground cinnamon
- 1 tsp maple syrup
- 1 tablespoon walnut halves
- 2 tsp coconut oil
- 1 Anjou pear spiralized with blade
- 1 cup almond milk
- ½ tsp vanilla extract

DIRECTIONS

1. In a saucepan boil water and add oats for another 10 minutes
2. In a skillet heat coconut oil over medium heat and add almond milk, pear noodles, cinnamon, maple syrup and vanilla extract
3. Stir to simmer for about 10-15 minutes
   4. In another skillet place walnuts and cook for 5-6 minutes, remove from pan when ready
   5. Place the oatmeal in a bowl and top with pear mixture and toasted walnuts

CHOCOLATE BREAD

Serves: *2*

Prep Time: *10*   Minutes

Cook Time: *30*   Minutes

Total Time: *40*   Minutes

INGREDIENTS

- Coconut oil
- 1 cup oat flour

- ½ cup almond flour
- 1 tablespoon flaxseeds
- 5 tablespoons water
- ½ cup almond milk
- 1 tsp baking powder
- 1 tsp baking soda
- 1 tsp vanilla extract
- ½ cup maple syrup
- 1 banana
- ½ cup cocoa powder

DIRECTIONS

1. Preheat oven to 300 F
2. Mix water with flax and water and set aside
3. In a bowl mash the banana and add remaining ingredients
4. Transfer the mixture to a loaf pan and bake for 40 minutes
5. Remove from the oven and let it cool
6. Slice the bread and serve

Serves: *2*

Prep Time: *10*   Minutes

Cook Time: *60*   Minutes

Total Time: *70*   Minutes

INGREDIENTS

- 1 cup hazelnut flour
- 1 peach
- 8 tablespoons water
- 6 tablespoons olive oil
- ¾ tsp salt
- 1 tsp cacao powder
- ½ tsp cinnamon
- 1 cup water
- ¼ tsp ginger
- ½ tablespoons coconut flakes
- 1 cup coconut flour
- 2 tablespoons flaxseeds
- 1 tablespoon cherries

DIRECTIONS

1. Preheat oven to 325 F

2. In a bowl mix water with flaxseeds

3. In another bowl mix all the ingredients, excepting coconut flakes and form a ball

4. Transfer the dough to a baking sheet with parchment paper

5. Sprinkle with coconut flakes and bake for 50 minutes

6. Remove and let it cool before serving

ALMOND BUTTER

Serves: **4**

Prep Time: **10** Minutes

Cook Time: **30** Minutes

Total Time: **40** Minutes

INGREDIENTS

- 1 cup pitted dates
- 2 bananas
- 1 cup almond flour
- 1 cup oats
- 2 tablespoons almond butter
- 2 tablespoons cherries
- 1 tsp sesame seeds

DIRECTIONS

1. In a food processor puree the dates until well combined
2. Add bananas and puree them also
3. Add oats, almond butter, almond flour, and puree until well combined
4. Transfer to the fridge for 25-30 minutes
5. Remove from fridge and add cherries and mix and also sesame seeds
6. Roll into small balls and place them on a baking sheet and bake for 20-25 minutes
7. Remove from oven and let them cool before serving

LEMON ZINGER BARS

Serves: *4*

Prep Time: *15*   Minutes

Cook Time: *35*   Minutes

Total Time: *50*   Minutes

INGREDIENTS

- 2 cups oats
- zest from 2 lemons

- 2/4 cup water
- 3 pitted dates chopped
- 2/4 cup apricots

DIRECTIONS

1. Preheat oven to 350 F
2. In a food processor add the oats and blend, pour the mixture into a bowl
3. Add the dates and apricots to the food processor
4. Add water and lemon juice and blend, let the mixture rest for 25-30 minutes
5. Bake for 30-35 minutes until golden brown and then remove from the oven
6. Remove from the pan onto a cutting board and cut into small bars
7. Store in a container for 1 week

Serves: *4*

Prep Time: *10*   Minutes

Cook Time: *20*   Minutes

Total Time: *30*   Minutes

INGREDIENTS

- ¾ cup pumpkin seeds
- 1 tablespoon hemp seeds
- 1 tsp sesame seeds
- ¼ cup carrot
- 1 tsp parsley
- ¼ tsp Chile powder
- 1/8 garlic
- ¼ tsp salt
- 1 tablespoons water
- ½ cup sunflower seeds

DIRECTIONS

1. Preheat oven to 325 F
2. In a blender place all the ingredients and blend
3. Add water and blend until a rough dough forms
4. Place the dough on a parchment paper

5. Use a pizza cutter to trim the edges and transfer to the oven
6. Bake for 15-20 minutes and remove from oven
7. Let it cool and serve

SWEET POTATO FLATBREAD

Serves: **4**

Prep Time: **25**   Minutes

Cook Time: **45**   Minutes

Total Time: **70**   Minutes

INGREDIENTS

- 1 sweet potato
- 2 tablespoons olive oil
- 1 tablespoon flaxseeds
- 2 tablespoons water
- 2 cups almond flour
- 1 tsp thyme
- 1 tsp chopped rosemary
- ½ tsp sea salt

DIRECTIONS

1. Preheat the oven to 325 F
2. Steam the sweet potato in a steamer basket over medium heat
3. In a bowl mix water with flaxseeds and set aside
4. In a bowl mash the sweet potatoes and add the remaining ingredients and mix
5. Transfer the mixture to a parchment lined baking sheet
6. Bake for 40 minutes or until golden brown
7. Remove from the oven and let it cool before serving

MANGO BEET SALAD

Serves: *4*

Prep Time: *20*   Minutes

Cook Time: *40*   Minutes

Total Time: *60*   Minutes

INGREDIENTS

- 5 beets
- 1 mango peeled
- 2 tablespoons walnuts

27

- 1 tablespoon coconut flakes
- 1 cup arugula
- 1 tablespoon almond oil
- juice from 1 lemon
- 1 pinch of salt

DIRECTIONS

1. Preheat the oven to 375 F
2. In a baking dish add the beets and roast for 35 minutes and add water, remove set aside
3. In another bowl mix the mango, walnuts, beets, arugula and coconut flakes
4. In a small bowl whisk lemon juice, sea salt, pepper, almond oil, pepper and salt
5. Drizzle the dressing over the salad and serve

Serves: *4*

Prep Time: *10*   Minutes

Cook Time: *30*   Minutes

Total Time: *40*   Minutes

INGREDIENTS

- Coconut oil
- 1 cup coconut milk
- 1 tablespoons vanilla extract
- 1 tablespoon maple syrup
- 1 cup while mulberries
- ½ tsp ground cinnamon
- 2 cups oats
- 2 tablespoons flaxseeds
- ¼ tsp salt
- ¼ tsp pumpkin pie spice
- ¼ tsp ground ginger

DIRECTIONS

1. Preheat oven to 325 F and grease a baking dish with coconut oil
2. Mix all the ingredients except cinnamon and transfer to a baking dish and sprinkle with cinnamon

3. Bake for 25-30 minutes, remove and let it cool
4. Cut into squares and serve

SESAME ALMOND COOKIES

Serves: **4**

Prep Time: **10**   Minutes

Cook Time: **20**   Minutes

Total Time: **30**   Minutes

INGREDIENTS

- 2 cups almond flour
- 2 tablespoons maple syrup
- 1 tablespoon coconut oil
- 3 tablespoons flaxseeds
- ½ tsp baking soda
- 1 tablespoon sesame seeds
- black pepper
- 1 pinch salt
- 1 pinch cinnamon

DIRECTIONS

1. Preheat oven to 325 F
2. In a bowl mix baking soda, almond flour, flaxseeds, sea salt and black pepper until well combined
3. Add coconut oil, maple syrup and vanilla extract and mix well
4. Add sesame seeds and cinnamon
5. Transfer to baking sheets by forming small cookies
6. Bake for 15-20 minutes and remove
7. Let it cool before serving

GLUTEN-FREE OATMEAL

Serves: *1*

Prep Time: *5*   Minutes

Cook Time: *10*   Minutes

Total Time: *15*   Minutes

INGREDIENTS

- 1/3 cup gluten free oats
- nourish snacks mocha mazing
- nourish snacks nutty nanas

DIRECTIONS

1. Cook oats following the indications on the package
2. Add almond milk with topping and serve

QUINOA CRANBERRY SALAD

Serves: 2

Prep Time: **10**   Minutes

Cook Time: **10**   Minutes

Total Time: **20**   Minutes

INGREDIENTS

- 1 cup quinoa
- 1 tablespoons cashews
- 1 tablespoon fresh basil
- 1 tablespoon vinegar
- 1 tablespoon olive oil
- 1 tsp orange juice
- ½ orange zest
- salt
- 1 red pepper
- 2 tablespoons cranberries

DIRECTIONS

1. Cook quinoa following the indications on the package
2. In a bowl toss quinoa with pepper, cashews, cranberries and basil
3. In another bowl whisk orange zest, salt, olive oil, vinegar, pepper and drizzle over quinoa salad

BLACK BEAN AND TAAHINI DIP

Serves: *1*

Prep Time: 5 Minutes

Cook Time: 5 Minutes

Total Time: *10* Minutes

INGREDIENTS

- 1 15 oz. black beans
- 1 tsp flax seeds
- sea salt
- ½ cup tahini sesame seeds

DIRECTIONS

1. In a food processor add all the ingredients and puree until smooth
2. Transfer to a bowl and serve

CHIA LEMON QUINOA

Serves: *2*

Prep Time: *10*   Minutes

Cook Time: *10*   Minutes

Total Time: *20*   Minutes

INGREDIENTS

- 1 cup quinoa
- 4 tablespoons maple syrup
- 3 tablespoons almonds
- 1 tablespoon chia seeds
- ½ tsp salt
- lemon zest
- 1 cup almond milk

DIRECTIONS

1. Cook quinoa following the indications on the package

2. Remove from heat and set aside

3. Add maple syrup, honey, chia seeds, almond milk, lemon zest and serve

GLUTEN-FREE QUINOA SWEET-PEA SALAD

Serves:	*3*
Prep Time:	*10* Minutes
Cook Time:	*10* Minutes
Total Time:	*20* Minutes

INGREDIENTS

- ½ cup quinoa
- 2 tablespoons parsley
- ¼ tsp orange zest
- ¼ tsp salt
- 1 bottle gluten-free beer
- 1/3 tsp cumin
- 2 tablespoons olive oil
- 1 red bell pepper

DIRECTIONS

1. Cook quinoa following the indications on the package
2. Remove and transfer to a bowl and set aside
3. Add the remaining ingredients and toss
4. Serve when ready

BUTTERNUT SQUASH WITH ALMOND BUTTER

Serves: *3*

Prep Time: *10* Minutes

Cook Time: *60* Minutes

Total Time: *70* Minutes

INGREDIENTS

- 2 tablespoons almond butter
- 1 butternut squash
- 1 pinch salt
- 1 pinch lemon zest

DIRECTIONS

1. Preheat oven to 325 F

2. In a baking dish place the squash and sprinkle with salt

3. Pour water into the baking dish and bake for 60 minutes

4. Remove from oven and drizzle with almond butter and lemon zest

5. Season with salt and pepper before serving

LUNCH

EGG SALAD

Serves: *2*

Prep Time: *10*   Minutes

Cook Time: *20*   Minutes

Total Time: *30*   Minutes

INGREDIENTS

- 5 eggs boiled and peeled
- 1 tablespoon mustard
- ½ tsp salt
- 2 tablespoons mayonnaise

DIRECTIONS

1. Cut the eggs in half and remove the yolks
2. In a bowl add all the ingredients and the yolks and mix everything
3. Spoon the mixture into the egg whites and serve

PICKLED BEETS

Serves: **4**

Prep Time: **10**   Minutes

Cook Time: **60**   Minutes

Total Time: **70**   Minutes

INGREDIENTS

- 1 bunch beets
- ¼ cup cider vinegar
- ¼ cup water
- 1 onion
- 1 clove garlic
- ¼ tsp salt
- 1 tablespoon honey

DIRECTIONS

1. In a saucepan add the beets and water and boil on high heat for 40-45 minutes

2. Drain and peel the beets and slice them

3. Put the beets back in the saucepan and add the rest of the ingredients except honey

4. Cook for 15 min, remove from heat and add honey

AVOCADO DIP

Serves:	2	
Prep Time:	5	Minutes
Cook Time:	10	Minutes
Total Time:	15	Minutes

INGREDIENTS

- 2 avocados
- ¼ cup mayonnaise
- ¼ tsp salt
- ½ tsp sesame oil
- 1 clove garlic
- 1 tablespoon chives

DIRECTIONS

1. Place all the ingredients in a blender and blend until smooth
2. Remove and serve

Serves: **2**

Prep Time: **10**   Minutes

Cook Time: **5**   Minutes

Total Time: **15**   Minutes

INGREDIENTS

- 1 cup frozen cherries
- ¼ tsp almond extract
- 1 tsp honey
- ¼ cup ice cubes
- 1 tsp flaxseed
- ¾ cup almond milk
- ¼ tsp vanilla

DIRECTIONS

1. In a blender add all the ingredients and blend until smooth
2. Pour into a glass and serve

EGGS WITH BEARNAISE SAUCE

Serves: *3*

Prep Time: *20*   Minutes

Cook Time: *20*   Minutes

Total Time: *40*   Minutes

INGREDIENTS

- 1 serving béarnaise sauce
- 2 cups water
- 3 eggs
- 1 tsp apple cider vinegar
- parsley
- 1 tablespoon ghee
- 1 shallot
- 1 clove garlic
- 1 lbs. baby spinach

DIRECTIONS

1. Prepare the sauce and set aside
2. In a pan heat the ghee and add garlic, shallot and sauté over medium heat
3. Add spinach and water and boil for 4-5 minutes and add vinegar when water is boiling
4. In a custard cup crack the eggs
5. Add the eggs and poach for 2-3 minutes
6. Divide the spinach on 3 plates and top with eggs

GREEN BEANS WITH MUSHROOMS

Serves: *4*

Prep Time: *10*   Minutes

Cook Time: *10*   Minutes

Total Time: *20*   Minutes

INGREDIENTS

- ½ lbs. green beans
- 1 shallot
- ¼ tsp thyme leaves
- ¼ tsp basil

- 1 tsp cider vinegar
- 1 clove garlic
- 3-ounces mushrooms
- ¼ tsp salt
- 1 tablespoon almonds
- 1 tablespoon olive oil

DIRECTIONS

1. Steam the beans for 4-5 minutes
2. In a pan add olive oil and shallot and sauce over medium heat for 2-3 minutes
3. Add garlic, mushrooms and green beans and sauté for 2-3 minutes
4. Stir in thyme, salt, basil and vinegar
5. Sprinkle sliced almonds over and serve

Serves: **4**

Prep Time: **10**   Minutes

Cook Time: **20**   Minutes

Total Time: **30**   Minutes

INGREDIENTS

- 2 cups cooked brown rice
- 2 ounces steamed green beans
- 1 cup bok choy
- 1 cup carrots

DIRECTIONS

1. On a plate place the rice and top with green beans, carrots and bok choy
2. Spoon vinaigrette over the vegetables and serve

Serves: *3*
Prep Time: *10*   Minutes

Cook Time: *10*   Minutes

Total Time: *20*   Minutes

INGREDIENTS

- 1 tsp olive oil
- 1 cup mushrooms
- 1 scallion
- 1 clove of garlic
- 1 tsp chopped herbs
- ¼ tsp salt
- 1 egg beaten

DIRECTIONS

1. In a pan add garlic, mushrooms and scallion over medium heat and cook for 2-3 minutes
2. Mix the egg with the herbs and pour the mixture into the pan
3. Cook for another 3-4 minutes

Serves: *3*

Prep Time: *10*   Minutes

Cook Time: *10*   Minutes

Total Time: *20*   Minutes

INGREDIENTS

- 1 cup almond flour
- ½ cup coconut
- 1 tablespoon honey
- 1 tablespoon coconut oil
- 1 tsp vanilla extract
- ¼ tsp almond extract
- 1 pinch salt

DIRECTIONS

1. Preheat oven to 325 F
2. Place all the ingredients in a blender and blend until smooth
3. Line a baking sheet with parchment paper and divide the dough into 9 portions
4. Bake for 10 minutes or until brown, remove and serve

Serves: *4*

Prep Time: *10*   Minutes

Cook Time: *45*   Minutes

Total Time: *55*   Minutes

INGREDIENTS

- 2 tablespoons olive oil
- 1 tsp salt
- 2 cups vegetable broth
- 1 stalk celery
- 6 oz. asparagus
- 1 tsp chopped dill
- 1 cup coconut milk
- 1 onion
- 1 clove garlic
- 1 carrot
- ¼ tsp chopped parsley

DIRECTIONS

1. In a saucepan add onions and sauté for 2-3 minutes over medium heat
2. Add asparagus, garlic, carrots and sauté for another 4-5 minutes

3. Add the remaining ingredients and bring to boil for 30-34 minutes
4. Remove from heat and let it cool
5. Puree the soup until smooth and serve

RICE PANCAKE

Serves: **4**

Prep Time: **10**   Minutes

Cook Time: **30**   Minutes

Total Time: **40**   Minutes

INGREDIENTS

- 1 tablespoon olive oil
- ¼ tsp salt
- ¼ tsp garlic powder
- 1 egg
- 1 cup brown rice
- 1 tsp chopped parsley
- 1 tsp chopped chives

DIRECTIONS

1. In a bowl mix all the ingredients
2. Pour the mixture into a frying pan over medium heat
3. Cook for 4-5 minutes
4. Remove and serve

ALMOND TIPALIA

Serves: *2*

Prep Time: *10*   Minutes

Cook Time: *10*   Minutes

Total Time: *20*   Minutes

INGREDIENTS

- 2/3 cup almond meal
- 4 tilapia filets
- 2 tablespoons coconut oil
- 1 tsp chopped parsley
- 1 clove garlic
- ½ tsp salt

DIRECTIONS

1. In a bowl mix herbs, salt and garlic
2. Coat both side of filet with the mixture
3. Refrigerate the fish for 30-40 minutes
4. Heat oil in a frying pan and cook the fish 5-6 minutes per side

ARTICHOKE LEK SOUP

Serves: **4**

Prep Time: **10** Minutes

Cook Time: **20** Minutes

Total Time: **30** Minutes

INGREDIENTS

- 1 tablespoon olive oil
- ½ cup almond milk
- ¼ tsp salt
- 1 tsp parsley
- 2 leeks
- 2 cloves garlic
- 1 can artichoke hearts
- 1 cup vegetable stock

DIRECTIONS

1. In a saucepan heat oil over medium heat
2. Sauté the leeks for 2-3 minutes and add garlic
3. Add the rest of the ingredients and bring to boil
4. Lover the heat and simmer for another 15-20 minutes
5. Remove and serve

COCONUT SMOOTHIE

Serves: **2**

Prep Time: **5** Minutes

Cook Time: **10** Minutes

Total Time: **15** Minutes

INGREDIENTS

- 1 cup coconut milk
- ¼ cup raspberries
- 1 tsp honey
- ¼ cup ice
- ¼ cup pomegranate

- ¼ cup blueberries

DIRECTIONS

1. In a blender add all the ingredients and blend until smooth
2. Pour into a glass and serve

ALMOND BUTTER

Serves: **2**

Prep Time: **10** Minutes

Cook Time: **10** Minutes

Total Time: **20** Minutes

INGREDIENTS

- 1 cup roasted almonds
- ¼ tsp salt

DIRECTIONS

1. In a blender place the ingredients and blend until smooth
2. Remove and serve

Serves: *4*

Prep Time: *10*   Minutes

Cook Time: *20*   Minutes

Total Time: *30*   Minutes

INGREDIENTS

- 1 lbs. flounder filet
- 1 tablespoon chopped shallots
- 1 clove garlic
- ¼ tsp chopped oregano
- parsley
- ½ tsp salt
- ½ cup mayonnaise
- 1 tsp mustard

DIRECTIONS

1. Preheat oven to broil
2. Mix all the ingredients (without parsley) and spread the mixture over the fish
3. Broil the fish for 10-12 minutes or until golden brown
4. Garnish with parsley and serve

Serves: **2**

Prep Time: **10** Minutes

Cook Time: **20** Minutes

Total Time: **30** Minutes

INGREDIENTS

- 2 lbs. green apples
- ¼ tsp salt
- 2 tsp honey
- 2/3 cup water
- ½ tsp cinnamon

DIRECTIONS

1. In a saucepan mix all the ingredients and bring to boil over medium heat
2. Cover the pot and lower the temperature
3. Cook for 20-25 minutes
4. Remove from heat and let it cool for 10-15 minutes
5. Stir in the honey and serve

Serves: **4**

Prep Time: **10** Minutes

Cook Time: **30** Minutes

Total Time: **40** Minutes

INGREDIENTS

- 2 cups shredded carrots
- ¼ tsp lemon thyme
- 1 tsp apple cider vinegar
- 1 tablespoon walnuts
- ½ cup mayonnaise
- 1 tsp honey
- 1 tsp chopped chives

DIRECTIONS

1. In a bowl mix all the ingredients
2. Refrigerate for 40-50 minutes, remove and serve

Serves: **2**

Prep Time: **10**   Minutes

Cook Time: **20**   Minutes

Total Time: **30**   Minutes

INGREDIENTS

RUB
- 1 tsp garlic powder
- ½ tsp oregano
- ½ tsp curry powder
- ¼ tsp ginger
- ½ tsp onion powder
- ½ tsp ground turmeric
- ½ tsp salt

FISH
- 2 salmon filets
- 1 small onion
- 1 tablespoon olive oil

DIRECTIONS

1. Preheat oven to 425 F
2. In a bowl mix all the ingredients for the rub and spread it over the salmon

56

3. Cook the fish for 10 minutes
4. Sauté the onion in the oil and place the sautéed onion
5. Remove and serve

GRILLED SALMON WITH HERB VINAIGRETTE

Serves: *2*

Prep Time: *10*   Minutes

Cook Time: *20*   Minutes

Total Time: *30*   Minutes

INGREDIENTS

SALMON
- 2 salmon filets
- 1 tsp olive oil
- salt
- pepper

GREENS
- 1 cup greens
- ½ cup chopped celery
- ¼ cup string beans
- 1 asparagus spears

57

- 1 tablespoon chopped nuts
- ½ cup shredded carrots
- 1 tablespoon dried cranberries

DIRECTIONS

1. Preheat the oven to broil
2. Brush the salmon filets with oil and season with salt
3. Broil the filets for 10 minutes
4. Mix all the ingredients for greens and pour ½ the vinaigrette over the greens
5. Plate the greens with grilled filet
6. Drizzle vinaigrette over the fish and serve

DINNER

BAKED ZUCCHINI

Serves: **4**

Prep Time: **10** Minutes

Cook Time: **20** Minutes

Total Time: **30** Minutes

INGREDIENTS

- 2 medium zucchini
- 2 cup shredded mozzarella cheese
- salt

DIRECTIONS

1. Slice zucchini into small pieces
2. Place flat into a cookie sheet
3. Sprinkle with salt
4. Bake for 15 minutes at 325 F
5. Remove ad sprinkle with cheese
6. Put it back in the oven for another 5 minutes
7. Remove and serve

Serves: *4*

Prep Time: *10*   Minutes

Cook Time: *60*   Minutes

Total Time: *70*   Minutes

INGREDIENTS

- 2 cups rice
- 3 cups chicken broth
- 1 tablespoon lime juice
- 2 4 oz. cans green chiles
- 1/3 cup cilantro
- 1 tsp oregano
- 1 tsp cumin
- 3 green onions

DIRECTIONS

1. In a pan mix all the ingredients
2. Bake until rice is done at 325 F
3. Remove and serve

Serves: *4*

Prep Time: *10*   Minutes

Cook Time: *10*   Minutes

Total Time: *40*   Minutes

INGREDIENTS

- 2 cups basil leaves
- 1 tsp olive oil
- ½ cup parmesan cheese
- ½ tsp salt
- ½ tsp ground pepper
- ½ cup walnuts

DIRECTIONS

1. Place all the ingredients in a blender and blend until smooth
2. Add olive oil in the pesto until is the right consistency
3. Remove and serve

Serves: **4**

Prep Time: **10** Minutes

Cook Time: **15** Minutes

Total Time: **25** Minutes

INGREDIENTS

- 2 cups cherry tomatoes
- ½ cup dried thyme
- 2 tablespoons olive oil
- ½ cup sweet onion
- ½ cup brown sugar

DIRECTIONS

1. In a pan heat olive oil and add onions
2. Sauce for 2-3 minutes and add tomatoes, thyme and sugar
3. Smash the tomatoes with a spoon
4. When ready remove from heat and serve

Serves: **4**

Prep Time: **20** Minutes

Cook Time: **30** Minutes

Total Time: **50** Minutes

INGREDIENTS

- 5 tablespoons butter
- 1 tsp salt
- 1 cup jake cheese
- 1 cup gruyere cheese
- ½ cup breadcrumbs
- 2 tablespoons parmesan cheese
- 2 cups macaroni dry
- ¼ cup purpose flour
- 2 cups milk
- ¼ tsp oregano
- 1 pinch red pepper

DIRECTIONS

1. Preheat oven to 375 F
2. Boil a large pot of water and cook until ready
3. In a pan melt butter and add flour and whisk to combine

4. Add milk and stir until smooth
5. Add seasoning and cheese and cook until each cheese is melted
6. Add pasta into the mixture
7. Sprinkle parmesan over top of pasta and serve

ROASTED BRUSEELS SPROUTS

Serves: *4*

Prep Time: *10*   Minutes

Cook Time: *10*   Minutes

Total Time: *20*   Minutes

INGREDIENTS

- 2 tablespoons olive oil
- 1 lb. Brussels sprouts
- ½ tsp salt
- ¼ tsp black pepper
- 2 tablespoons butter
- 1 tablespoon maple syrup

DIRECTIONS

1. Preheat oven to 400 F
2. Coat Brussels sprouts with olive oil and salt
3. Pour sprouts onto baking sheet and roast for 12-15 minutes
4. Flip them while roasting
5. In a saucepan melt butter and cook until brown
6. Remove from heat and add maple syrup

CARAMELIZED ONION AND BACON

Serves: *4*

Prep Time: *10* Minutes

Cook Time: *30* Minutes

Total Time: *40* Minutes

INGREDIENTS

- 1 lbs. green beans
- 4 slices bacon
- 1 onion
- 1 tsp sugar
- 3 tablespoons butter
- Salt

DIRECTIONS

1. In a pan add butter and cook onion until brown
2. Add sugar, balsamic vinegar and stir to combine
3. Transfer onions to a bowl and melt butter and add beans
4. Cook until brown for 9-10 minutes
5. Add in caramelized onions, bacon and salt

CORNCAKE

Serves: **4**

Prep Time: **10** Minutes

Cook Time: **20** Minutes

Total Time: **30** Minutes

INGREDIENTS

- ½ cup butter
- ½ cup sugar
- 1 tablespoon whipping cream
- 1/3 tssp salt
- ½ tsp baking powder
- ½ cup masa harina
- 1/3 cup water

- 1 cup creamed corn
- ½ cup corn

DIRECTIONS

1. Preheat oven to 325 F
2. Beat butter until creamy and add water and masa harina and mix
3. Add cornmeal, sugar, corn, baking powder and salt
4. Pour the mixture into an iron pan
5. Bake for 20-25 minutes, remove and serve

TERIYAKI BURGER

Serves: *4*

Prep Time: *10*   Minutes

Cook Time: *20*   Minutes

Total Time: *30*   Minutes

INGREDIENTS

- 1 lbs. ground beep
- 2 tablespoons teriyaki sauce

- 1 tablespoon honey
- 1 tsp salt
- ¾ tsp ginger
- 1 clove garlic minced
- 4 hamburger buns
- lettuce leaves
- tomato slices

DIRECTIONS

1. Mix first 6 ingredients into 4 patties
2. Cook patties on grill
3. Place on bun, lettuce, tomato and condiments
4. Serve when ready

Serves: **2**

Prep Time: **5** Minutes

Cook Time: **5** Minutes

Total Time: **10** Minutes

INGREDIENTS

- 1 chicken breast
- ¼ cup dressing
- ½ cup bbq sauce
- 1 cup tortilla strips
- ½ cup bbq sauce
- 5 cups romaine lettuce
- 1 cup corn
- 1 cup black beans
- ½ cup cheese
- 1 tomato
- 1 avocado

DIRECTIONS

1. Cook the chicken and cover with bbq sauce
2. Mix corn, black beans, romaine lettuce, avocado, cheese and tomato

3. Mix together bbq sauce and dressing and add to salad
4. Serve when ready

STRAWBERRY SALAD

Serves: **2**

Prep Time: **5** Minutes

Cook Time: **5** Minutes

Total Time: **10** Minutes

INGREDIENTS

- ½ lb. romaine lettuce
- ½ cup pneapple
- ½ cup strawberries
- ½ cup blueberries
- 1 can oranges
- ½ cup pecans

DIRECTIONS

1. Slice fruit and mix with lettuce and serve

Serves: 2

Prep Time: 5   Minutes

Cook Time: 10   Minutes

Total Time: 15   Minutes

INGREDIENTS

- 4 strips bacon
- ½ cup tomatoes
- ½ cup mayonnaise
- 3 tablespoons balsamic vinegar
- 3 onions
- 1 lb. tube pasta
- 1 lb. chicken cooked and shredded
- 3 cups spinach

DIRECTIONS

1. In a bowl add balsamic vinegar and mayonnaise and whisk well
2. In another bowl mix onion, pasta, bacon, chicken spinach and tomatoes
3. Add mayonnaise mixture and toss to combine

Serves: *2*

Prep Time: *10*   Minutes

Cook Time: *60*   Minutes

Total Time: *70*   Minutes

INGREDIENTS

- 6 oz. bow tie pasta
  ### DRESSING

- 1 cup oil
- 1/3 cup teriyaki sauce
- 1 5 oz. can water chestnuts
- 2 onions
- ¼ tsp salt
- ¼ tsp pepper
- 8 oz. spinach
- 1 cup craisins
- 1 11 oz can oranges
- 2 tablespoons sesame seeds
- 1 cup peanuts
- 1/3 cup white vinegar
- 5 tablespoons sugar

DIRECTIONS

1. In a blender add all the dressing ingredients and blend
2. Combine remaining dressing and pasta and marinade for 1-2 hours
3. Add pasta and liquid and toss well
4. Remove and serve

BUTTERNUT SQUASH SOUP

Serves: **4**

Prep Time: **10** Minutes

Cook Time: **30** Minutes

Total Time: **40** Minutes

INGREDIENTS

- 2 tablespoons butter
- 24 oz. cubed butternut squash
- 2 cups chicken broth
- 1 pinch cumin
- salt
- ¼ onion
- 1 clove garlic
- ¼ tsp thyme

DIRECTIONS

1. Coat squash with olive oil and place it on a baking sheet
2. Broil for 10-12 minutes
3. In a pan melt butter and add onion, garlic and thyme
4. Add squash and chicken broth and cook for 10-12 minutes
5. Add pepper, salt and cumin
6. Remove from heat and puree the mixture

TACO SOUP

Serves: 2

Prep Time: *10*   Minutes

Cook Time: *30*   Minutes

Total Time: *40*   Minutes

INGREDIENTS

- 1 lb. hamburger
- 1 16 oz. can tomato sauce
- 2 16 oz. can red kidney beans
- taco seasoning
- ½ cup onion
- 3 cups water

- 2 26 oz. cans tomatoes

DIRECTIONS

1. **Combine all ingredients and simmer for 15-20 minutes**
2. **Top with cheese and sliced olives**

PUMPKIN CHILI

Serves: *2*
Prep Time: *10*   Minutes

Cook Time: *30*   Minutes

Total Time: *40*   Minutes

INGREDIENTS

- 2 tablespoons olive oil
- 1 small onion
- 2 cups chicken stock
- 1 tablespoon chili powder
- 1 tsp cumin
- ½ tsp salt
- 1 can kidney beans
- 1 green bell pepper

- 1 jalapeno seed
- 1 clove garlic
- 1 lb. ground chicken
- 1 can 15 oz. tomatoes
- 1 15 oz. can pumpkin puree

DIRECTIONS

1. In a pot heat oil and add pepper, onion and garlic
2. Sauté until tender and add turkey, pumpkin, tomatoes, chili powder, cumin and salt
3. Reduce heat and add beans
4. Simmer for 30 minutes
5. Remove from heat and serve

Serves: **4**

Prep Time: **10** Minutes

Cook Time: **240** Minutes

Total Time: **250** Minutes

INGREDIENTS

- 1 lb. chicken breast
- ¼ tsp pepper
- 1 cup frozen peas
- 1 cup frozen corn
- ½ tsp thyme
- 3 cups chicken broth
- ½ cup flour
- 1 tsp garlic minced
- 1 tsp salt
- 1 tsp oregano
- ½ cup onion
- 1 cup carrots

DIRECTIONS

1. In a slow cooker add all the ingredients except the peas
2. Cook for 4 hours or until chicken is ready

3. Remove chicken and shred and return to the cooker with the peas and cook for another 30 minutes

4. Use a cookie cutter and cut shapes from the pie crust

5. Bake according to directions on package and use them to garnish the soup

TOMATO TORTELLINI SOUP

Serves: **4**

Prep Time: **10** Minutes

Cook Time: **20** Minutes

Total Time: **30** Minutes

INGREDIENTS

- ½ cup chopped tomatoes
- 6 oz. cheese tortellini
- ½ cup onion
- 1 cup carrot
- 1 tsp sugar
- ½ cup whipping cream
- Parmesan cheese
- basil
- 1 tablespoon tomato paste

- 1 tsp garlic minced
- 4 cups chicken broth
- 1 cup tomatoes
- 1 tsp salt

DIRECTIONS

1. In a pot mix tomato with oil, onion, carrots, tomato paste and garlic
2. Sauté for 3-4 minutes and add salt, pepper and chicken broth
3. Simmer for 15-17 minutes
4. Puree soup with a blender until smooth
5. Cook tortellini in boiling water and add cream to soup
6. Garnish with parmesan, basil and serve

Serves: **4**

Prep Time: **10** Minutes

Cook Time: **20** Minutes

Total Time: **30** Minutes

INGREDIENTS

- 2 cups mashed sweet potatoes
- 1 tsp cumin
- ½ cup onion
- 1 tablespoon butter
- ½ tsp salt
- 1 tablespoon cilantro
- ¼ cup coconut milk
- 2 cups chicken broth
- ½ tsp red pepper flakes

DIRECTIONS

1. In a pan over medium heat sauté onion in butter until soft
2. Add onions into sweet potatoes and chicken broth
3. Simmer for 10-15 minutes on high heat and season with salt, cumin and red pepper
4. Add coconut milk and cook for another 5-10 minutes

5.   Garnish with cilantro and serve

TURKEY SOUP

Serves: *4*

Prep Time: *10*   Minutes

Cook Time: *20*   Minutes

Total Time: *30*   Minutes

INGREDIENTS

- 1 cup onion
- 1 tsp cumin
- 1 tsp salt
- ¼ tsp salt
- ¼ tsp pepper
- 1 15 oz. can black beans
- 1 11 oz. can whole kernel corn
- 1 10 oz. can tomatoes
- 1 tsp chili powder
- 1 tsp canola oil
- 1 tsp garlic
- 3 cups chicken broth
- 2 cups turkey chopped

- grated cheese

DIRECTIONS

1. In a pan sauce onion with garlic over medium heat
2. Add the rest of ingredients and sauté for another 2-3 minutes
3. Boil and simmer for 15-20 minutes
4. Serve with grated cheese

DESSERT

GRANOLA COOKIES

Serves: 2

Prep Time: 5   Minutes

Cook Time: 10   Minutes

Total Time: 15   Minutes

INGREDIENTS

- ¾ cuppb
- ½ cup oats
- ½ cup brown sugar

- 2 cups granola
- 3 oz chocolate
- 2/3 cup honey

DIRECTIONS

1. In a blender add granola and blend until smooth
2. Lay out a piece of wax paper
3. In a saucepan mix peanut butter, honey and brown sugar
4. Bring to boil over medium heat for 4-5 minutes
5. Turn off heat and pour over granola mixture
6. Scoop onto wax paper and top with chocolate

Serves: **2**

Prep Time: 5   Minutes

Cook Time: 5   Minutes

Total Time: **10**   Minutes

INGREDIENTS

- 8 cups chex cereal
- 1 cup pretzel twists
- 1 cup mixed nuts
- ¼ cup melted coconut oil
- ½ coconut amino
- 1 tsp salt

DIRECTIONS

1. In a bowl mix all the ingredients together and serve

Serves: **20**

Prep Time: **10**   Minutes

Cook Time: **10**   Minutes

Total Time: **20**   Minutes

INGREDIENTS

- ¼ cup coconut oil
- ¾ cup chocolate chips
- ¼ cup brown sugar
- 1 egg
- 1 cup shredded coconut
- 1 tsp salt
- 1 cup oats

DIRECTIONS

1. Preheat oven to 325 F and line a baking sheet with parchment paper
2. In a bowl mix eggs, coconut oil and sugar until smooth
3. Add salt, oats and coconut stir well
4. Scoop the dough and shape into a ball and place on the cookie sheet
5. Bake for 15-20 minutes
6. When ready, remove and serve

Serves: **4**

Prep Time: **10** Minutes

Cook Time: **20** Minutes

Total Time: **30** Minutes

INGREDIENTS

- ¼ cup coconut oil
- 1 10 oz. marshmallows
- 4 cups rice cereal

DIRECTIONS

1. In a pan mix marshmallow with coconut oil over medium heat until melted
2. When mixture is smooth add rice cereal and mix
3. Pour into pan and cool for an hour
4. Remove and cut into squares

Serves: **24**

Prep Time: **10**   Minutes

Cook Time: **20**   Minutes

Total Time: **30**   Minutes

INGREDIENTS

- 1 cup peanut butter
- ¼ cup M&M's
- ¾ cup brown sugar
- 1 tablespoons maple syrup
- 1 cup oats¼ cup M&M's
- ¼ cup chocolate chips
- ¼ cup chocolate chips
- 4 tablespoons coconut oil

DIRECTIONS

1. On the counter place a wax paper and store where you will store peanut butter balls
2. In a bowl mix brown sugar, peanut butter, coconut oil, maple syrup until smooth
3. Add oats and mix
4. Add chocolate chips and M&M's and stir well
5. Form small balls and place them on the wax paper

Serves: **4**

Prep Time: **10** Minutes

Cook Time: **50** Minutes

Total Time: **60** Minutes

INGREDIENTS

- 1 cup chocolate chips
- ¾ cup oat flour
- ¼ tsp salt
- ¼ cup chocolate chips
- ¾ cup coconut oil
- 1 cup raw sugar
- 3 eggs
- 1 tsp vanilla

DIRECTIONS

1. In a bowl mix coconut oil and chocolate chips and microwave for 1 minute and put aside
2. Preheat oven to 325 F and and line a baking pan with foil
3. In a bowl mix eggs and sugar until smooth and add chocolate mixture and vanilla and mix well
4. Fold in the oat flour, chocolate chips, salt and pour into the pan

5. Bake for 45-50 minutes, remove and serve

BLUEBERRY BANANA MUFFINS

Serves: **4**

Prep Time: **10**   Minutes

Cook Time: **30**   Minutes

Total Time: **40**   Minutes

INGREDIENTS

- 2 bananas
- ½ tsp baking soda
- ½ tsp cinnamon
- ½ tsp salt
- 1 cup cassava flour
- ¾ cup blueberries
- 2 eggs
- ½ cup olive oil
- ½ cup coconut sugar

DIRECTIONS

1. Preheat oven to 325 F and line a muffin tin

2. Place wet ingredients and sugar in blender and blend until smooth

3. In a bowl mix dry ingredients and pour into blender and blend until smooth

4. Add blueberries and stir

5. Pour mixture into muffin cups

6. Bake until golden brown for 20-25 minutes

7. Remove and serve

COCONUT OIL COOKIES

Serves: *4*

Prep Time: *10*   Minutes

Cook Time: *10*   Minutes

Total Time: *20*   Minutes

INGREDIENTS

- 3 cup oats
- 1 cup sugar
- ½ cup cocoa powder
- ¼ tsp salt
- 1 tsp vanilla
- ½ cup coconut oil

- ¼ cup peanut butter
- ¼ cup cashew milk

DIRECTIONS

1. In a saucepan mix, peanut butter, cashew milk, coconut oil, sugar, salt and cocoa powder and cook over medium heat for 4-5 minutes
2. Add vanilla and oats to mixture and cook for another 2-3 minutes
3. Scoop into a wax paper and let it cool before serving

GLUTEN FREE INSTANT POT OATMEAL

Serves: *2*

Prep Time: *10* Minutes

Cook Time: *10* Minutes

Total Time: *20* Minutes

INGREDIENTS

- 2 cups gluten free oats
- 2 cups water
- 2 tablespoons coconut vinegar

- 3 cups milk
- ¼ tsp sat

DIRECTIONS

1. In a bowl mix oats, water, vinegar and cover for 24 hours
2. Add oats mixture to the instant pot and add milk and salt
3. Cook for 4-5 minutes, remove and serve

BANANA BREAD COOKIES

Serves: **4**

Prep Time: **10**   Minutes

Cook Time: **10**   Minutes

Total Time: **20**   Minutes

INGREDIENTS

- 1 cup purpose flour
- 1 tsp vanilla extract
- 1 tablespoon canola oil
- ¼ cup chocolate chips
- ¼ tsp baking soda

- 1 tsp baking powder
- ½ banana
- 1 tablespoon agave syrup
- 2 tablespoons applesauce

DIRECTIONS

1. Preheat oven to 325 F
2. In a bowl mix baking soda, baking powder and flour
3. In another bowl smash a banana and add applesauce, agave syrup, vanilla extract and canola oil
4. Add wet ingredients to the dry ingredients and mix until it forms a dough
5. Add chocolate chips and mix together
6. Scoop the dough onto parchment paper covered with baking sheets
7. Bake for 10 minutes and remove when ready

Serves: **2**

Prep Time: **10**   Minutes

Cook Time: **10**   Minutes

Total Time: **20**   Minutes

INGREDIENTS

- 1 cup oats
- 1 tsp vanilla extract
- pinch of salt
- 3 tablespoons water
- 2 tablespoons cacao powder
- 2 tablespoons hemp seeds
- 1 tablespoon chia seeds

DIRECTIONS

1. Place the ingredients into a blender and blend until smooth
2. Add water and blend again
3. Roll into small balls and refrigerate

Serves:	*12*
Prep Time:	*10* Minutes
Cook Time:	*10* Minutes
Total Time:	*20* Minutes

INGREDIENTS

- ¼ cup cashew butter
- 1 cup vanilla protein powder
- ¼ cup almond flour
- 2 tablespoons orange juice

DIRECTIONS

1. In a bowl mix orange juice with cashew
2. Stir until combined completely and add protein powder and almond flour
3. Roll dough into balls and store in refrigerator

95

Serves: *12*

Prep Time: *10*   Minutes

Cook Time: *20*   Minutes

Total Time: *30*   Minutes

INGREDIENTS

- 1 cup oats
- ½ cup maple syrup
- ½ cup peanut butter
- ¼ cup shredded coconut
- ¼ cup hemp hearts
- ½ cup chocolate chips

DIRECTIONS

1. In a bowl add shredded coconut, hemp hears, oats and chocolate chips and whisk to combine
2. Add maple syrup and peanut butter and mix until well combined
3. Scoop a tablespoon of mixture and roll into balls and set aside
4. Repeat the process and refrigerate the balls

Serves: **12**

Prep Time: **10** Minutes

Cook Time: **30** Minutes

Total Time: **40** Minutes

INGREDIENTS

- 1 cup shredded carrots
- ½ cup oats
- ¾ cup desiccated coconut
- 1/3 cup almonds
- 2 tablespoons hemp seeds
- 1 tsp cinnamon
- 1 tsp nutmeg
- 1/3 tsp ginger
- ¼ tsp salt
- 1 tablespoon coconut oil
- 1 tsp tapioca flour
- ¼ cup vegan chocolate

DIRECTIONS

1. In a bowl put ¼ of coconut
2. In a blender add all the ingredients and blend until smooth

3. Scoop out a tablespoon of the batter and roll into a ball
4. Drizzle the chocolate on top and refrigerate

PEACH COBBLER SMOOTHIE

Serves: *1*

Prep Time: *5*   Minutes

Cook Time: *5*   Minutes

Total Time: *10*   Minutes

INGREDIENTS

- 1 cup oat milk
- ½ cup water
- 1 cup frozen peaches
- 1 tablespoon rolled oats
- ¼ tsp vanilla extract
- ¼ tsp cinnamon
- ¼ tsp nutmeg

DIRECTIONS

1. Place all the ingredients in a blender and blend until smooth

2. Pour in a glass and serve

CHERRY COCONUT SMOOTHIE

Serves: *2*
Prep Time: *10*   Minutes

Cook Time: *10*   Minutes

Total Time: *20*   Minutes

INGREDIENTS

- 2 cups frozen blueberries
- 1 cup baby spinach
- 1 16-ounce coconut milk
- red layer
- 1 cup frozen cherries
- 1 date
- 1 tablespoon hemp seeds

DIRECTIONS

1. Place all the ingredients in a blender and blend until smooth
2. Pour in a glass and serve

Serves: **2**

Prep Time: **5** Minutes

Cook Time: **5** Minutes

Total Time: **10** Minutes

INGREDIENTS

- 1 banana
- ½ cup frozen blackberries
- ¼ cup water
- ½ cup lettuce
- ½ cup coconut milk
- 1 tablespoon chia seeds
- 2 ice cubes

DIRECTIONS

1. Place all the ingredients in a blender and blend until smooth
2. Pour in a glass and serve

Serves: 2

Prep Time: 5 Minutes

Cook Time: 5 Minutes

Total Time: 10 Minutes

INGREDIENTS

- 5-ounces water
- 2 tsp turmeric
- 1 tsp ginger
- ¼ tsp black pepper
- 1 cup carrots
- 1 cup pineapple
- ¼ cup cashews
- 2 fresh dates

DIRECTIONS

1. Place all the ingredients in a blender and blend until smooth
2. Pour in a glass and serve

Serves:	**2**
Prep Time:	**5** Minutes
Cook Time:	**5** Minutes
Total Time:	**10** Minutes

INGREDIENTS

- 1 cup almond milk
- ¼ tsp ginger
- ½ tsp nutmeg
- ¼ tsp cloves
- 1 frozen banana
- ½ cup rolled oats
- 2 tsp black strap molasses
- ¼ tsp cinnamon

DIRECTIONS

1. Place all the ingredients in a blender and blend until smooth
2. Pour in a glass and serve

Serves: 2

Prep Time: 5   Minutes

Cook Time: 5   Minutes

Total Time: 10   Minutes

INGREDIENTS

- 1 cup almond milk
- ¼ tsp cinnamon
- 2 ice cubes
- 1 orange
- 1 baked potato
- ¼ tsp ginger

DIRECTIONS

1. Place all the ingredients in a blender and blend until smooth
2. Pour in a glass and serve

LYME DISEASE COOKBOOK

40+ Side dishes, Salad and Pasta recipes designed for Lyme Disease

ZUCCHINI PIZZA

Serves: **6-8**

Prep Time: **10**   Minutes

Cook Time: **15**   Minutes

Total Time: **25**   Minutes

INGREDIENTS

- 1 pizza crust
- ½ cup tomato sauce
- ¼ black pepper
- 1 cup zucchini slices
- 1 cup mozzarella cheese
- 1 cup olives

DIRECTIONS

1. Spread tomato sauce on the pizza crust
2. Place all the toppings on the pizza crust
3. Bake the pizza at 425 F for 12-15 minutes
4. When ready remove pizza from the oven and serve

Serves: **6-8**

Prep Time: **10**   Minutes

Cook Time: **15**   Minutes

Total Time: **25**   Minutes

INGREDIENTS

- 1 pizza crust
- ½ cup tomato sauce
- ¼ black pepper
- 1 cup salami slices
- 1 cup mozzarella cheese
- 1 cup olives

DIRECTIONS

1. Spread tomato sauce on the pizza crust
2. Place all the toppings on the pizza crust
3. Bake the pizza at 425 F for 12-15 minutes
4. When ready remove pizza from the oven and serve

Serves: *6-8*

Prep Time: *10*   Minutes

Cook Time: *15*   Minutes

Total Time: *25*   Minutes

INGREDIENTS

- 1 pizza crust
- ½ cup tomato sauce
- ¼ black pepper
- 1 lb. cooked chicken breast
- 1 cup mozzarella cheese
- 1 cup olives

DIRECTIONS

1. Spread tomato sauce on the pizza crust
2. Place all the toppings on the pizza crust
3. Bake the pizza at 425 F for 12-15 minutes
4. When ready remove pizza from the oven and serve

Serves: **6-8**

Prep Time: **10** Minutes

Cook Time: **15** Minutes

Total Time: **25** Minutes

INGREDIENTS

- 1 pizza crust
- ½ cup tomato sauce
- ¼ black pepper
- ¼ cup zucchini slices
- ¼ cup olives
- ¼ cup tomatoes
- ¼ cucumber
- 1 cup mozzarella cheese
- 1 cup olives

DIRECTIONS

1. Spread tomato sauce on the pizza crust
2. Place all the toppings on the pizza crust
3. Bake the pizza at 425 F for 12-15 minutes
4. When ready remove pizza from the oven and serve

Serves: **4**

Prep Time: **10**   Minutes

Cook Time: **20**   Minutes

Total Time: **30**   Minutes

INGREDIENTS

- 1 tablespoon olive oil
- 1 lb. broccoli
- ¼ red onion
- ½ cup all-purpose flour
- ¼ tsp salt
- ¼ tsp pepper
- 1 can vegetable broth
- 1 cup heavy cream

DIRECTIONS

1. In a saucepan heat olive oil and sauté broccoli until tender
2. Add remaining ingredients to the saucepan and bring to a boil
3. When all the vegetables are tender transfer to a blender and blend until smooth
4. Pour soup into bowls, garnish with parsley and serve

Serves: **4**

Prep Time: **10**   Minutes

Cook Time: **20**   Minutes

Total Time: **30**   Minutes

INGREDIENTS

- 1 tablespoon olive oil
- 1 lb. zucchini
- ¼ red onion
- ½ cup all-purpose flour
- ¼ tsp salt
- ¼ tsp pepper
- 1 can vegetable broth
- 1 cup heavy cream

DIRECTIONS

1. In a saucepan heat olive oil and sauté zucchini until tender
2. Add remaining ingredients to the saucepan and bring to a boil
3. When all the vegetables are tender transfer to a blender and blend until smooth
4. Pour soup into bowls, garnish with parsley and serve

Serves: **4**

Prep Time: **10**   Minutes

Cook Time: **20**   Minutes

Total Time: **30**   Minutes

INGREDIENTS

- 1 tablespoon olive oil
- 1 lb. cauliflower
- ¼ red onion
- ½ cup all-purpose flour
- ¼ tsp salt
- ¼ tsp pepper
- 1 can vegetable broth
- 1 cup heavy cream

DIRECTIONS

1. In a saucepan heat olive oil and sauté cauliflower until tender
2. Add remaining ingredients to the saucepan and bring to a boil
3. When all the vegetables are tender transfer to a blender and blend until smooth
4. Pour soup into bowls, garnish with parsley and serve

Serves: **4**

Prep Time: **10** Minutes

Cook Time: **20** Minutes

Total Time: **30** Minutes

INGREDIENTS

- 1 tablespoon olive oil
- 1 lb. cucumber
- ¼ red onion
- ½ cup all-purpose flour
- ¼ tsp salt
- ¼ tsp pepper
- 1 can vegetable broth
- 1 cup heavy cream

DIRECTIONS

1. In a saucepan heat olive oil and sauté cucumber until tender
2. Add remaining ingredients to the saucepan and bring to a boil
3. When all the vegetables are tender transfer to a blender and blend until smooth
4. Pour soup into bowls, garnish with parsley and serve

Serves: *4*

Prep Time: *10*   Minutes

Cook Time: *15*   Minutes

Total Time: *25*   Minutes

INGREDIENTS

- 1 onion
- 2 chicken breasts
- 2 tablespoons unsalted butter
- 2 eggs
- 2 cups cooked rice
- 2 cups cheese
- 1 cup parmesan cheese
- 2 cups cooked broccoli

DIRECTIONS

1. Sauté the veggies and set aside
2. Preheat the oven to 425 F
3. Transfer the sautéed veggies to a baking dish, add remaining ingredients to the baking dish
4. Mix well, add seasoning and place the dish in the oven
5. Bake for 12-15 minutes or until slightly brown

Serves: **4**

Prep Time: **10**   Minutes

Cook Time: **15**   Minutes

Total Time: **25**   Minutes

INGREDIENTS

- 1 tablespoon olive oil
- 1 cup red bell peppers
- 1 cup red onion
- 1 jalapeno pepper
- 1 cup corn kernels
- 1 can red beans
- 1 can tomatoes
- 1 cup cheddar cheese
- ½ cup seasoning mixture

DIRECTIONS

1. Sauté the veggies and set aside
2. Preheat the oven to 425 F
3. Transfer the sautéed veggies to a baking dish, add remaining ingredients to the baking dish
4. Mix well, add seasoning and place the dish in the oven

5. Bake for 12-15 minutes or until slightly brown
6. When ready remove from the oven and serve

CARROT CASSEROLE

Serves: *4*

Prep Time: *10*   Minutes

Cook Time: *15*   Minutes

Total Time: *25*   Minutes

INGREDIENTS

- 1 onion
- 1 cup parmesan cheese
- 1 tsp smoked paprika
- 1 lb. carrots
- 3 sticks celery
- 1 red pepper
- 1 can tomatoes
- ½ lb. lentils
- 1 yellow pepper

DIRECTIONS

1. Sauté the veggies and set aside
2. Preheat the oven to 425 F
3. Transfer the sautéed veggies to a baking dish, add remaining ingredients to the baking dish
4. Mix well, add seasoning and place the dish in the oven
5. Bake for 12-15 minutes or until slightly brown
6. When ready remove from the oven and serve

BEEF CASSEROLE

Serves: *4*

Prep Time: *10*   Minutes

Cook Time: *15*   Minutes

Total Time: *25*   Minutes

INGREDIENTS

- 1 onion
- 2 celery sticks
- 2 carrots
- 3-4 bay leaves

- 1 tablespoon olive oil
- 3-4 tablespoons flour
- 2 lb. stewing beef
- 2 beef stock cubes

DIRECTIONS

1. Sauté the veggies and set aside
2. Preheat the oven to 425 F
3. Transfer the sautéed veggies to a baking dish, add remaining ingredients to the baking dish
4. Mix well, add seasoning and place the dish in the oven
5. Bake for 12-15 minutes or until slightly brown
6. When ready remove from the oven and serve

Serves: *1*

Prep Time: 5   Minutes

Cook Time: 5   Minutes

Total Time: *10*   Minutes

INGREDIENTS

- 6 oz. goat cheese
- ½ cup ricotta cheese
- 1 scallion
- 1 tsp lemon zest
- 1 tablespoons lemon juice
- 1 tsp black pepper

DIRECTIONS

1. In a blender add all ingredients together
2. Blend until smooth
3. Serve when ready

Serves: *1*

Prep Time: 5   Minutes

Cook Time: 5   Minutes

Total Time: *10*   Minutes

INGREDIENTS

- 2 oz. cranberries
- ¼ cup swerve
- 1 cinnamon stick
- 1 orange zest
- 1 tablespoon vanilla extract

DIRECTIONS

1. In a blender add all ingredients together
2. Blend until smooth
3. Serve when ready

Serves: **1**

Prep Time: 5 Minutes

Cook Time: 5 Minutes

Total Time: **10** Minutes

INGREDIENTS

- 2 tablespoons olive oil
- 1 onion
- 2 garlic cloves
- 1 can tomatoes
- 2 tablespoons vinegar
- Basil leaves
- ¼ tsp salt

DIRECTIONS

1. In a blender add all ingredients together
2. Blend until smooth
3. Serve when ready

Serves: *1*

Prep Time: 5   Minutes

Cook Time: 5   Minutes

Total Time: *10*   Minutes

INGREDIENTS

- 2 tablespoons olive oil
- 2 tablespoons fermented black beans
- 1 tablespoon garlic
- 1 tablespoon soy sauce
- 1 tablespoon rice wine
- 1 tsp cornstarch

DIRECTIONS

1. In a blender add all ingredients together
2. Blend until smooth
3. Serve when ready

Serves: **2**

Prep Time: **10** Minutes

Cook Time: **20** Minutes

Total Time: **30** Minutes

INGREDIENTS

- 1 cup edamame
- 1 tablespoon olive oil
- ½ red onion
- 2 eggs
- ¼ tsp salt
- 2 oz. cheddar cheese
- 1 garlic clove
- ¼ tsp dill

DIRECTIONS

1. In a bowl whisk eggs with salt and cheese
2. In a frying pan heat olive oil and pour egg mixture
3. Add remaining ingredients and mix well
4. Serve when ready

Serves: **2**

Prep Time: **10**   Minutes

Cook Time: **20**   Minutes

Total Time: **30**   Minutes

INGREDIENTS

- 2-3 garlic cloves
- 1 tablespoon olive oil
- ½ red onion
- 2 eggs
- ¼ tsp salt
- 2 oz. cheddar cheese
- 1 garlic clove
- ¼ tsp dill

DIRECTIONS

1. In a bowl whisk eggs with salt and cheese
2. In a frying pan heat olive oil and pour egg mixture
3. Add remaining ingredients and mix well
4. Serve when ready

Serves: **2**

Prep Time: **10**   Minutes

Cook Time: **20**   Minutes

Total Time: **30**   Minutes

INGREDIENTS

- 1 cup black beans
- 1 tablespoon olive oil
- ½ red onion
- 2 eggs
- ¼ tsp salt
- 2 oz. cheddar cheese
- 1 garlic clove
- ¼ tsp dill

DIRECTIONS

1. In a bowl whisk eggs with salt and cheese
2. In a frying pan heat olive oil and pour egg mixture
3. Add remaining ingredients and mix well
4. Serve when ready

Serves:	*3-4*
Prep Time:	*10* Minutes
Cook Time:	*20* Minutes
Total Time:	*30* Minutes

INGREDIENTS

- 2 delicata squashes
- 2 tablespoons olive oil
- 1 tsp curry powder
- 1 tsp salt

DIRECTIONS

1. Preheat the oven to 400 F
2. Cut everything in half lengthwise
3. Toss everything with olive oil and place onto a prepared baking sheet
4. Roast for 18-20 minutes at 400 F or until golden brown
5. When ready remove from the oven and serve

Serves: **3-4**

Prep Time: **10**   Minutes

Cook Time: **20**   Minutes

Total Time: **30**   Minutes

INGREDIENTS

- 1 cucumber
- 2 tablespoons olive oil
- 1 tsp curry powder
- 1 tsp salt

DIRECTIONS

1. Preheat the oven to 400 F
2. Cut everything in half lengthwise
3. Toss everything with olive oil and place onto a prepared baking sheet
4. Roast for 18-20 minutes at 400 F or until golden brown
5. When ready remove from the oven and serve

Serves: **3-4**

Prep Time: **10**   Minutes

Cook Time: **20**   Minutes

Total Time: **30**   Minutes

INGREDIENTS

- 1 carrot
- 2 tablespoons olive oil
- 1 tsp curry powder
- 1 tsp salt

DIRECTIONS

1. Preheat the oven to 400 F
2. Cut everything in half lengthwise
3. Toss everything with olive oil and place onto a prepared baking sheet
4. Roast for 18-20 minutes at 400 F or until golden brown
5. When ready remove from the oven and serve

Serves: **2**

Prep Time: **10** Minutes

Cook Time: **20** Minutes

Total Time: **30** Minutes

INGREDIENTS

- 1 lb. brussels sprouts
- 1 tablespoon olive oil
- 1 tablespoon parmesan cheese
- 1 tsp garlic powder
- 1 tsp seasoning

DIRECTIONS

1. Preheat the oven to 425 F
2. In a bowl toss everything with olive oil and seasoning
3. Spread everything onto a prepared baking sheet
4. Bake for 8-10 minutes or until crisp
5. When ready remove from the oven and serve

Serves: *2*

Prep Time: *10*   Minutes

Cook Time: *20*   Minutes

Total Time: *30*   Minutes

INGREDIENTS

- 1 lb. kale
- 1 tablespoon olive oil
- 1 tablespoon parmesan cheese
- 1 tsp garlic powder
- 1 tsp seasoning

DIRECTIONS

1. Preheat the oven to 425 F
2. In a bowl toss everything with olive oil and seasoning
3. Spread everything onto a prepared baking sheet
4. Bake for 8-10 minutes or until crisp
5. When ready remove from the oven and serve

Serves: *2*

Prep Time: *10*   Minutes

Cook Time: *20*   Minutes

Total Time: *30*   Minutes

INGREDIENTS

- 1 lb. potatoes
- 1 tablespoon olive oil
- 1 tablespoon parmesan cheese
- 1 tsp garlic powder
- 1 tsp seasoning

DIRECTIONS

1. Preheat the oven to 425 F
2. In a bowl toss everything with olive oil and seasoning
3. Spread everything onto a prepared baking sheet
4. Bake for 8-10 minutes or until crisp
5. When ready remove from the oven and serve

PASTA

SIMPLE SPAGHETTI

Serves:	*2*	
Prep Time:	*5*	Minutes
Cook Time:	*15*	Minutes
Total Time:	*20*	Minutes

INGREDIENTS

- 10 oz. spaghetti
- 2 eggs
- ½ cup parmesan cheese
- 1 tsp black pepper
- Olive oil
- 1 tsp parsley
- 2 cloves garlic

DIRECTIONS

1. In a pot boil spaghetti (or any other type of pasta), drain and set aside
2. In a bowl whish eggs with parmesan cheese
3. In a skillet heat olive oil, add garlic and cook for 1-2 minutes
4. Pour egg mixture and mix well

5. Add pasta and stir well

6. When ready garnish with parsley and serve

SALMON PASTA

Serves: 2

Prep Time: 5   Minutes

Cook Time: 15   Minutes

Total Time: 20   Minutes

INGREDIENTS

- 1 lb. spaghetti
- 1 red onion
- 2 cloves garlic
- 1 cup heavy cream
- ½ lb. salmon
- 1 tablespoon dill
- Parmesan cheese

DIRECTIONS

1. In a pot boil spaghetti (or any other type of pasta), drain and set aside

2. Place all the ingredients for the sauce in a pot and bring to a simmer

3. Add pasta and mix well

4. When ready garnish with parmesan cheese and serve

CACIO E PEPE

Serves: 2

Prep Time: 5   Minutes

Cook Time: 15   Minutes

Total Time: 20   Minutes

INGREDIENTS

-   1 lb. pasta
-   1 butter stick
-   1 tablespoon olive oil
-   1 cup pecorino
-   1 cup parmesan cheese

DIRECTIONS

1. In a pot boil spaghetti (or any other type of pasta), drain and set aside
2. Place all the ingredients for the sauce in a pot and bring to a simmer
3. Add pasta and mix well
4. When ready garnish with parmesan cheese and serve

LIME SHRIMP PASTA

Serves: **2**

Prep Time: **5** Minutes

Cook Time: **15** Minutes

Total Time: **20** Minutes

INGREDIENTS

- 14 cup olive oil
- 1 tablespoon lime juice
- 1 tsp cumin
- 1 lb. shrimp
- 1 lb. spaghetti
- 2 cloves arlic

- ¼ cup cilantro
- ¼ tsp red pepper flakes

DIRECTIONS

1. In a pot boil spaghetti (or any other type of pasta), drain and set aside
2. Place all the ingredients for the sauce in a pot and bring to a simmer
3. Add pasta and mix well
4. When ready garnish with parmesan cheese and serve

CHICKEN CARBONARA

Serves: 2

Prep Time: 5   Minutes

Cook Time: 15   Minutes

Total Time: 20   Minutes

INGREDIENTS

- 10 oz. fettuccine
- 3-4 slices bacon

- 2-3 garlic cloves
- 1 lb. cooked chicken breast
- 2 eggs
- 1 cup parmesan cheese
- ¼ cup parsley

DIRECTIONS

1. In a pot boil spaghetti (or any other type of pasta), drain and set aside
2. Place all the ingredients for the sauce in a pot and bring to a simmer
3. Add pasta and mix well
4. When ready garnish with parmesan cheese and serve

SALAD

MORNING SALAD

Serves: **2**

Prep Time: **5**   Minutes

Cook Time: **5**   Minutes

Total Time: **10**   Minutes

INGREDIENTS

- 1 onion
- 1 tsp cumin
- 1 tablespoon olive oil
- 1 avocado
- ¼ lb. cooked lentils
- 1 oz. walnuts
- Coriander
- ¼ lb. feta cheese
- Salad dressing of choice
- 8-10 baby carrots

DIRECTIONS

1. In a bowl combine all ingredients together and mix well
2. Add dressing and serve

Serves: **2**

Prep Time: **5**   Minutes

Cook Time: **5**   Minutes

Total Time: **10**   Minutes

INGREDIENTS

- 1 tsp tamari
- 1 tsp curry powder
- 1 garlic clove
- 1 tsp honey
- 1 tablespoon peanut butter
- 1 tablespoon chili sauce
- 1 tablespoon lime juice
- ½ cucumber
- 1 shallot
- 2 cooked chicken breasts

DIRECTIONS

1. In a bowl combine all ingredients together and mix well
2. Add dressing and serve

Serves: 2

Prep Time: 5   Minutes

Cook Time: 5   Minutes

Total Time: 10   Minutes

INGREDIENTS

- 1 onion
- 1 tablespoon apple cider vinegar
- 2 handful rocket leaves
- 2 cooked beetroots
- 2 oz. halloumi
- 2 oz. pomegranate seeds
- 2 tablespoons pumpkin seeds

DIRECTIONS

1. In a bowl combine all ingredients together and mix well
2. Add dressing and serve

Serves: 2

Prep Time: 5 Minutes

Cook Time: 5 Minutes

Total Time: **10** Minutes

INGREDIENTS

- 1 basil
- 1 bunch parsley
- 2 lb. roasted potatoes
- 2-3 tablespoons olive oil
- 1 garlic clove

DIRECTIONS

1. In a bowl combine all ingredients together and mix well
2. Add dressing and serve

Serves: **2**

Prep Time: **5**   Minutes

Cook Time: **5**   Minutes

Total Time: *10*   Minutes

INGREDIENTS

- 1 onion
- ½ lb. tomatoes
- 2 oz. watercress
- 1 tsp wine vinegar
- 2 tablespoons olive oil
- 1 tsp mustard

DIRECTIONS

1. In a bowl combine all ingredients together and mix well
2. Add dressing and serve

Serves: *2*

Prep Time: *5*   Minutes

Cook Time: *5*   Minutes

Total Time: *10*   Minutes

INGREDIENTS

- 1 red onion
- 2-3 hard boiled eggs
- 1 tsp tahini
- 1 tsp cumin
- 1 can fava beans
- 1 tomato

DIRECTIONS

1. In a bowl combine all ingredients together and mix well
2. Add dressing and serve

Serves: *2*

Prep Time: 5   Minutes

Cook Time: 5   Minutes

Total Time: *10*   Minutes

INGREDIENTS

- 2 garlic cloves
- 1 shallot
- 2 tablespoons capers
- 2 cooked salmon fillets
- 2 tablespoon olive oil
- ¼ cup olives

DIRECTIONS

1. In a bowl combine all ingredients together and mix well
2. Add dressing and serve

Serves: **2**

Prep Time: **5**   Minutes

Cook Time: **5**   Minutes

Total Time: **10**   Minutes

INGREDIENTS

- ½ lb. bulgur wheat
- ½ lb. cooked edamame
- 2 red peppers
- ¼ lb. radishes
- 2 oz. almonds
- 2 tablespoons olive oil

DIRECTIONS

1. In a bowl combine all ingredients together and mix well
2. Add dressing and serve

Serves: *2*

Prep Time: *5*   Minutes

Cook Time: *5*   Minutes

Total Time: *10*   Minutes

INGREDIENTS

- 1 tsp balsamic vinegar
- 1 garlic clove
- 1 tablespoon olive oil
- ¼ cup basil
- ¼ cup olive oil
- 2 hard boiled eggs
- ½ lb. green beans
- ¼ red onion
- ¼ cup olives

DIRECTIONS

1. In a bowl combine all ingredients together and mix well
2. Add dressing and serve

Serves: **2**

Prep Time: **5**   Minutes

Cook Time: **5**   Minutes

Total Time: **10**   Minutes

INGREDIENTS

- 3 oz. lentils
- ½ lb. cauliflower florets
- 2 tablespoons olive oil
- 1 carrot
- 2 celery sticks
- 2 garlic cloves
- ¼ lb. tomatoes
- ½ red onion

DIRECTIONS

1. In a bowl combine all ingredients together and mix well
2. Add dressing and serve

LYME DISEASE COOKBOOK

40+ Pancakes, muffins and Cookies
recipes designed for Lyme Disease

MUSHROOM OMELETTE

Serves: **1**

Prep Time: **5** Minutes

Cook Time: **10** Minutes

Total Time: **15** Minutes

INGREDIENTS

- 2 eggs
- ¼ tsp salt
- ¼ tsp black pepper
- 1 tablespoon olive oil
- ¼ cup cheese
- ¼ tsp basil
- 1 cup mushrooms

DIRECTIONS

1. In a bowl combine all ingredients together and mix well
2. In a skillet heat olive oil and pour the egg mixture
3. Cook for 1-2 minutes per side
4. When ready remove omelette from the skillet and serve

Serves: *1*

Prep Time: 5   Minutes

Cook Time: *10*   Minutes

Total Time: *15*   Minutes

INGREDIENTS

- 2 eggs
- ¼ tsp salt
- ¼ tsp black pepper
- 1 tablespoon olive oil
- ¼ cup cheese
- ¼ tsp basil

DIRECTIONS

1. In a bowl combine all ingredients together and mix well
2. In a skillet heat olive oil and pour the egg mixture
3. Cook for 1-2 minutes per side
4. When ready remove omelette from the skillet and serve

Serves: **1**

Prep Time: **5**   Minutes

Cook Time: **10**   Minutes

Total Time: **15**   Minutes

INGREDIENTS

- 2 eggs
- ¼ tsp salt
- ¼ tsp black pepper
- 1 tablespoon olive oil
- ¼ cup cheese
- ¼ tsp basil
- 1 cup cabbage

DIRECTIONS

1. In a bowl combine all ingredients together and mix well
2. In a skillet heat olive oil and pour the egg mixture
3. Cook for 1-2 minutes per side
4. When ready remove omelette from the skillet and serve

Serves: *1*

Prep Time: *5*   Minutes

Cook Time: *10*   Minutes

Total Time: *15*   Minutes

INGREDIENTS

- 2 eggs
- ¼ tsp salt
- ¼ tsp black pepper
- 1 tablespoon olive oil
- ¼ cup cheese
- ¼ tsp basil
- 8-10 oz. bacon

DIRECTIONS

1. In a bowl combine all ingredients together and mix well
2. In a skillet heat olive oil and pour the egg mixture
3. Cook for 1-2 minutes per side
4. When ready remove omelette from the skillet and serve

Serves: **1**

Prep Time: **5**   Minutes

Cook Time: **10**   Minutes

Total Time: **15**   Minutes

INGREDIENTS

-   2 eggs
-   ¼ tsp salt
-   ¼ tsp black pepper
-   1 tablespoon olive oil
-   ¼ cup cheese
-   1 tablespoon basil

DIRECTIONS

1. In a bowl combine all ingredients together and mix well
2. In a skillet heat olive oil and pour the egg mixture
3. Cook for 1-2 minutes per side
4. When ready remove omelette from the skillet and serve

TOMATO OMELETTE

Serves:	*1*
Prep Time:	*5* Minutes
Cook Time:	*10* Minutes
Total Time:	*15* Minutes

INGREDIENTS

- 2 eggs
- ¼ tsp salt
- ¼ tsp black pepper
- 1 tablespoon olive oil
- ¼ cup cheese
- ¼ tsp basil
- 3-4 tomato slices

DIRECTIONS

1. In a bowl combine all ingredients together and mix well
2. In a skillet heat olive oil and pour the egg mixture
3. Cook for 1-2 minutes per side
4. When ready remove omelette from the skillet and serve

Serves: *1*

Prep Time: *5* Minutes

Cook Time: *5* Minutes

Total Time: *10* Minutes

INGREDIENTS

- 1 cup corn cereal
- 1 cup rice cereal
- ¼ cup cocoa cereal
- ¼ cup rice cakes

DIRECTIONS

1. In a bowl combine all ingredients together
2. Serve with milk

Serves: *1*

Prep Time: *5* Minutes

Cook Time: *5* Minutes

Total Time: *10* Minutes

INGREDIENTS

- 1 cup corn cereal
- 1 cup rice cereal
- ¼ cup cocoa cereal
- ¼ cup rice cakes

DIRECTIONS

1. In a bowl combine all ingredients together
2. Serve with milk

Serves: **1**

Prep Time: 5 Minutes

Cook Time: 5 Minutes

Total Time: **10** Minutes

INGREDIENTS

- 1 tsp cinnamon
- 1 cup dried fruits
- 1 cup corn cereal
- 1 cup dried cherries
- 1 cup almond milk

DIRECTIONS

1. In a bowl combine all ingredients together
2. Serve with milk

Serves: *1*

Prep Time: *5*   Minutes

Cook Time: *5*   Minutes

Total Time: *10*   Minutes

INGREDIENTS

- ½ cup corn cereal
- 1 cup rice cereal
- ½ cup coconut flakes
- 1 cup berries
- 1 cup milk

DIRECTIONS

1. In a bowl combine all ingredients together
2. Serve with milk

Serves: **1**

Prep Time: 5   Minutes

Cook Time: 5   Minutes

Total Time: **10**   Minutes

INGREDIENTS

- ½ cup dried raisins
- ½ cup dried pecans
- ¼ cup almonds
- 1 cup coconut milk
- 1 tsp cinnamon

DIRECTIONS

1. In a bowl combine all ingredients together
2. Serve with milk

Serves: *2*

Prep Time: *5*   Minutes

Cook Time: *15*   Minutes

Total Time: *20*   Minutes

INGREDIENTS

- ¼ cup egg substitute
- 1 muffin
- 1 turkey sausage patty
- 1 tablespoon cheddar cheese

DIRECTIONS

1. In a skillet pour egg and cook on low heat
2. Place turkey sausage patty in a pan and cook for 4-5 minutes per side
3. On a toasted muffin place the cooked egg, top with a sausage patty and cheddar cheese
4. Serve when ready

Serves: *1*

Prep Time: 5   Minutes

Cook Time: 5   Minutes

Total Time: *10*   Minutes

INGREDIENTS

- 2 bread slices
- 6 bacon slices
- 2 fried eggs
- 1 tsp black pepper
- ½ avocado

DIRECTIONS

1. Slightly toast the bread slices
2. Place all the ingredients on a bread slice
3. Top with the other bread slice
4. Toast again until golden brown
5. Serve when ready

Serves: *1*

Prep Time: 5 Minutes

Cook Time: 5 Minutes

Total Time: *10* Minutes

INGREDIENTS

- 2 bread slices
- 1 lb. cooked beef
- ¼ cup BBQ sauce
- 2 slices cheddar cheese

DIRECTIONS

1. Slightly toast the bread slices
2. Place all the ingredients on a bread slice
3. Top with the other bread slice
4. Toast again until golden brown
5. Serve when ready

Serves: *1*

Prep Time: *5* Minutes

Cook Time: *5* Minutes

Total Time: *10* Minutes

INGREDIENTS

- 2 bread slices
- 2 fried eggs
- 1 tablespoon parmesan cheese
- 1 pinch salt
- 1 pinch black pepper
- 2 slices bacon
- 2 slices gouda cheese

DIRECTIONS

1. Slightly toast the bread slices
2. Place all the ingredients on a bread slice
3. Top with the other bread slice
4. Toast again until golden brown
5. Serve when ready

Serves: *1*

Prep Time: 5   Minutes

Cook Time: 5   Minutes

Total Time: *10*   Minutes

INGREDIENTS

- 2 bread slices
- 4 slices bacon
- 2 fried eggs
- 2 slices cheese
- ¼ cup guacamole

DIRECTIONS

1. Slightly toast the bread slices
2. Place all the ingredients on a bread slice
3. Top with the other bread slice
4. Toast again until golden brown
5. Serve when ready

Serves: *1*

Prep Time: 5   Minutes

Cook Time: 5   Minutes

Total Time: *10*   Minutes

INGREDIENTS

- 2 bread slices
- ¼ tsp red pepper flakes
- 1 tsp salt
- 1 tablespoon mayonnaise
- ¼ tsp paprika
- 1 cup cooked kale

DIRECTIONS

1. Slightly toast the bread slices
2. Place all the ingredients on a bread slice
3. Top with the other bread slice
4. Toast again until golden brown
5. Serve when ready

Serves: 2

Prep Time: 5   Minutes

Cook Time: 30   Minutes

Total Time: 35   Minutes

INGREDIENTS

- 1 tsp vanilla extract
- 1 tablespoon honey
- 1 lb. rolled oats
- 2 tablespoons sesame seeds
- ¼ lb. almonds
- ¼ lb. berries

DIRECTIONS

1. Preheat the oven to 325 F
2. Spread the granola onto a baking sheet
3. Bake for 12-15 minutes, remove and mix everything
4. Bake for another 12-15 minutes or until slightly brown
5. When ready remove from the oven and serve

Serves: **2**

Prep Time: **5**   Minutes

Cook Time: **30**   Minutes

Total Time: **35**   Minutes

INGREDIENTS

- 1 tsp orange zest
- 1 tsp brown sugar
- 3 cups rolled oats
- 1 cup almonds
- 1 tsp cinnamon
- 2 tablespoons honey
- 2 tablespoons orange juice

DIRECTIONS

1. Preheat the oven to 325 F
2. Spread the granola onto a baking sheet
3. Bake for 12-15 minutes, remove and mix everything
4. Bake for another 12-15 minutes or until slightly brown
5. When ready remove from the oven and serve

Serves: 2

Prep Time: 5   Minutes

Cook Time: 30   Minutes

Total Time: 35   Minutes

INGREDIENTS

- 1 tsp orange zest
- 1 tsp brown sugar
- 1 cup pecans
- ¼ cup raisins
- 2 cups oats
- 1 tsp cinnamon
- 1 cup cranberries

DIRECTIONS

1. Preheat the oven to 325 F
2. Spread the granola onto a baking sheet
3. Bake for 12-15 minutes, remove and mix everything
4. Bake for another 12-15 minutes or until slightly brown
5. When ready remove from the oven and serve

Serves: **2**

Prep Time: **5** Minutes

Cook Time: **30** Minutes

Total Time: **35** Minutes

INGREDIENTS

- 2 cups oats
- ¼ cup peanuts
- ¼ cup almonds
- ¼ cup chia seeds
- ¼ cup maple syrup
- 1 tsp vanilla extract
- ¼ cup coconut flakes

DIRECTIONS

1. Preheat the oven to 325 F
2. Spread the granola onto a baking sheet
3. Bake for 12-15 minutes, remove and mix everything
4. Bake for another 12-15 minutes or until slightly brown
5. When ready remove from the oven and serve

Serves: 2

Prep Time: 5   Minutes

Cook Time: 30   Minutes

Total Time: 35   Minutes

INGREDIENTS

- ½ lb. pecans
- ½ lb. walnuts
- 2 tsp vanilla essence
- 1 lb. rolled oats

DIRECTIONS

1. Preheat the oven to 325 F
2. Spread the granola onto a baking sheet
3. Bake for 12-15 minutes, remove and mix everything
4. Bake for another 12-15 minutes or until slightly brown
5. When ready remove from the oven and serve

CHERRY GRANOLA

Serves: **2**

Prep Time: **5** Minutes

Cook Time: **30** Minutes

Total Time: **35** Minutes

INGREDIENTS

- 1 lb. rolled oats
- ¼ cup coconut flakes
- ¼ lb. almonds
- ½ lb. dried cherries
- 2 tablespoons maple syrup
- 1 tsp cinnamon

DIRECTIONS

1. Preheat the oven to 325 F
2. Spread the granola onto a baking sheet
3. Bake for 12-15 minutes, remove and mix everything
4. Bake for another 12-15 minutes or until slightly brown
5. When ready remove from the oven and serve

PANCAKES

BANANA PANCAKES

Serves: *4*

Prep Time: *10*   Minutes

Cook Time: *20*   Minutes

Total Time: *30*   Minutes

INGREDIENTS

- 1 cup whole wheat flour
- ¼ tsp baking soda
- ¼ tsp baking powder
- 1 cup mashed banana
- 2 eggs
- 1 cup milk

DIRECTIONS

1. In a bowl combine all ingredients together and mix well
2. In a skillet heat olive oil
3. Pour ¼ of the batter and cook each pancake for 1-2 minutes per side
4. When ready remove from heat and serve

Serves: **4**

Prep Time: **10**   Minutes

Cook Time: **20**   Minutes

Total Time: **30**   Minutes

INGREDIENTS

- 1 cup whole wheat flour
- ¼ tsp baking soda
- ¼ tsp baking powder
- 2 eggs
- 1 cup milk

DIRECTIONS

1. In a bowl combine all ingredients together and mix well
2. In a skillet heat olive oil
3. Pour ¼ of the batter and cook each pancake for 1-2 minutes per side
4. When ready remove from heat and serve

Serves: **4**

Prep Time: **10** Minutes

Cook Time: **20** Minutes

Total Time: **30** Minutes

INGREDIENTS

- 1 cup whole wheat flour
- ¼ tsp baking soda
- ¼ tsp baking powder
- 1 cup dried cherries
- 2 eggs
- 1 cup milk

DIRECTIONS

1. In a bowl combine all ingredients together and mix well
2. In a skillet heat olive oil
3. Pour ¼ of the batter and cook each pancake for 1-2 minutes per side
4. When ready remove from heat and serve

Serves: **4**

Prep Time: **10** Minutes

Cook Time: **20** Minutes

Total Time: **30** Minutes

INGREDIENTS

- 1 cup whole wheat flour
- ¼ tsp baking soda
- ¼ tsp baking powder
- 1 cup mashed strawberries
- 2 eggs
- 1 cup milk

DIRECTIONS

1. In a bowl combine all ingredients together and mix well
2. In a skillet heat olive oil
3. Pour ¼ of the batter and cook each pancake for 1-2 minutes per side
4. When ready remove from heat and serve

Serves: *4*

Prep Time: *10*   Minutes

Cook Time: *20*   Minutes

Total Time: *30*   Minutes

INGREDIENTS

- 1 cup whole wheat flour
- ¼ tsp baking soda
- ¼ tsp baking powder
- 1 cup mashed pumpkin
- 2 eggs
- 1 cup milk

DIRECTIONS

1. In a bowl combine all ingredients together and mix well
2. In a skillet heat olive oil
3. Pour ¼ of the batter and cook each pancake for 1-2 minutes per side
4. When ready remove from heat and serve

Serves: **4**

Prep Time: **10**   Minutes

Cook Time: **20**   Minutes

Total Time: **30**   Minutes

INGREDIENTS

- 1 cup whole wheat flour
- ¼ tsp baking soda
- ¼ tsp baking powder
- 1 cup mashed peanuts
- 2 eggs
- 1 cup milk

DIRECTIONS

1. In a bowl combine all ingredients together and mix well
2. In a skillet heat olive oil
3. Pour ¼ of the batter and cook each pancake for 1-2 minutes per side
4. When ready remove from heat and serve

BREAKFAST COOKIES

Serves: *8-12*

Prep Time: 5   Minutes

Cook Time: *15*   Minutes

Total Time: *20*   Minutes

INGREDIENTS

- 1 cup rolled oats
- ¼ cup applesauce
- ½ tsp vanilla extract
- 3 tablespoons chocolate chips
- 2 tablespoons dried fruits
- 1 tsp cinnamon

DIRECTIONS

1. Preheat the oven to 325 F
2. In a bowl combine all ingredients together and mix well
3. Scoop cookies using an ice cream scoop
4. Place cookies onto a prepared baking sheet
5. Place in the oven for 12-15 minutes or until the cookies are done
6. When ready remove from the oven and serve

Serves: *8-12*

Prep Time: 5   Minutes

Cook Time: 15   Minutes

Total Time: 20   Minutes

INGREDIENTS

- 2 cups flour
- 1 cup rolled oats
- ¼ cup applesauce
- ½ cup honey
- 2 eggs
- 1 cup dried raisins
- ½ tsp vanilla extract

DIRECTIONS

1. Preheat the oven to 325 F
2. In a bowl combine all ingredients together and mix well
3. Scoop cookies using an ice cream scoop
4. Place cookies onto a prepared baking sheet
5. Place in the oven for 12-15 minutes or until the cookies are done
6. When ready remove from the oven and serve

Serves: *8-12*

Prep Time: 5   Minutes

Cook Time: 15   Minutes

Total Time: 20   Minutes

INGREDIENTS

- 2 cups oats
- 1 cup coconut flour
- 1 tsp cinnamon
- 1 tsp baking soda
- ½ cup honey
- 2 eggs
- 1 tsp vanilla extract

DIRECTIONS

1. Preheat the oven to 325 F
2. In a bowl combine all ingredients together and mix well
3. Scoop cookies using an ice cream scoop
4. Place cookies onto a prepared baking sheet
5. Place in the oven for 12-15 minutes or until the cookies are done
6. When ready remove from the oven and serve

Serves: *8-12*

Prep Time: 5   Minutes

Cook Time: *15*   Minutes

Total Time: *20*   Minutes

INGREDIENTS

- 2 cups coconut flour
- 2 cups chocolate chips
- 2 eggs
- 1 tsp vanilla essence
- 1 cup oats
- 1 tsp baking powder
- 2 tablespoons maple syrup

DIRECTIONS

1. Preheat the oven to 325 F
2. In a bowl combine all ingredients together and mix well
3. Scoop cookies using an ice cream scoop
4. Place cookies onto a prepared baking sheet
5. Place in the oven for 12-15 minutes or until the cookies are done
6. When ready remove from the oven and serve

Serves:	*8-12*
Prep Time:	*5* Minutes
Cook Time:	*15* Minutes
Total Time:	*20* Minutes

INGREDIENTS

- 1 cup oats
- 1 cup almond flour
- ¼ cup brown sugar
- 1 tsp baking powder
- 1 banana
- 1 egg

DIRECTIONS

1. Preheat the oven to 325 F
2. In a bowl combine all ingredients together and mix well
3. Scoop cookies using an ice cream scoop
4. Place cookies onto a prepared baking sheet
5. Place in the oven for 12-15 minutes or until the cookies are done
6. When ready remove from the oven and serve

Serves:	*8-12*	
Prep Time:	*5*	Minutes
Cook Time:	*15*	Minutes
Total Time:	*20*	Minutes

INGREDIENTS

- 1 cup oats
- 1 cup coconut flour
- 2 tablespoons brown sugar
- 1 cup dried cherries
- 1 tsp baking powder
- 1 banana
- 1 egg

DIRECTIONS

1. Preheat the oven to 325 F
2. In a bowl combine all ingredients together and mix well
3. Scoop cookies using an ice cream scoop
4. Place cookies onto a prepared baking sheet
5. Place in the oven for 12-15 minutes or until the cookies are done
6. When ready remove from the oven and serve

MUFFINS

SIMPLE MUFFINS

Serves:	*8-12*	
Prep Time:	*10*	Minutes
Cook Time:	*20*	Minutes
Total Time:	*30*	Minutes

INGREDIENTS

- 2 eggs
- 1 tablespoon olive oil
- 1 cup milk
- 2 cups whole wheat flour
- 1 tsp baking soda
- ¼ tsp baking soda
- 1 cup pumpkin puree
- 1 tsp cinnamon
- ¼ cup molasses

DIRECTIONS

1. In a bowl combine all dry ingredients
2. In another bowl combine all dry ingredients
3. Combine wet and dry ingredients together

4. Pour mixture into 8-12 prepared muffin cups, fill 2/3 of the cups

5. Bake for 18-20 minutes at 375 F

6. When ready remove from the oven and serve

SUNSHINE MUFFINS

Serves: **8-12**

Prep Time: **10**   Minutes

Cook Time: **20**   Minutes

Total Time: **30**   Minutes

INGREDIENTS

- ¼ cup brown sugar
- zest of 1 orange
- 1 cup almond flour
- 1 cup rolled oats
- 1 tsp baking powder
- 1 cup orange juice
- 2 eggs

DIRECTIONS

1. In a bowl combine all dry ingredients
2. In another bowl combine all dry ingredients
3. Combine wet and dry ingredients together
4. Pour mixture into 8-12 prepared muffin cups, fill 2/3 of the cups
5. Bake for 18-20 minutes at 375 F
6. When ready remove from the oven and serve

Serves: **8-12**

Prep Time: **10** Minutes

Cook Time: **20** Minutes

Total Time: **30** Minutes

INGREDIENTS

- 2 cups coconut flour
- 1 tsp baking powder
- 1 tsp cinnamon
- ¼ cup sugar
- 2 eggs
- 1 cup pumpkin puree
- ¼ cup sunflower seeds
- ¼ cup molasses

DIRECTIONS

1. In a bowl combine all dry ingredients
2. In another bowl combine all dry ingredients
3. Combine wet and dry ingredients together
4. Pour mixture into 8-12 prepared muffin cups, fill 2/3 of the cups
5. Bake for 18-20 minutes at 375 F, remove and serve

Serves: **8-12**

Prep Time: **10**   Minutes

Cook Time: **20**   Minutes

Total Time: **30**   Minutes

INGREDIENTS

- ½ cup brown sugar
- juice from 1 lemon
- zest from 1 lemon
- 1 cup coconut flour
- 1 cup oats
- 1 tsp baking soda
- 3 eggs
- 1 tablespoon poppy seeds

DIRECTIONS

1. In a bowl combine all dry ingredients
2. In another bowl combine all dry ingredients
3. Combine wet and dry ingredients together
4. Pour mixture into 8-12 prepared muffin cups, fill 2/3 of the cups
5. Bake for 18-20 minutes at 375 F, remove and serve

Serves: *8-12*

Prep Time: *10*   Minutes

Cook Time: *20*   Minutes

Total Time: *30*   Minutes

INGREDIENTS

- 2 eggs
- 1 cup cornmeal
- 2 tablespoons sugar
- 1 tsp baking powder
- 1 tsp baking soda
- 1 cup buttermilk
- ½ cup corn kernels
- 1 tsp cilantro

DIRECTIONS

1. In a bowl combine all dry ingredients
2. In another bowl combine all dry ingredients
3. Combine wet and dry ingredients together
4. Pour mixture into 8-12 prepared muffin cups, fill 2/3 of the cups
5. Bake for 18-20 minutes at 375 F, remove and serve

LYME DISEASE COOKBOOK

40+ Smoothies, Dessert and Breakfast
Recipes designed for Lyme Disease

BREAKFAST

BEANS OMELETTE

Serves: *1*

Prep Time: *5*   Minutes

Cook Time: *10*   Minutes

Total Time: *15*   Minutes

INGREDIENTS

- 2 eggs
- ¼ tsp salt
- ¼ tsp black pepper
- 1 tablespoon olive oil
- ¼ cup cheese
- ¼ tsp basil
- 1 cup beans

DIRECTIONS

1. In a bowl combine all ingredients together and mix well
2. In a skillet heat olive oil and pour the egg mixture
3. Cook for 1-2 minutes per side
4. When ready remove omelette from the skillet and serve

Serves: **1**

Prep Time: **5** Minutes

Cook Time: **10** Minutes

Total Time: **15** Minutes

INGREDIENTS

- 2 eggs
- ¼ tsp salt
- ¼ tsp black pepper
- 1 tablespoon olive oil
- ¼ cup cheese
- ¼ tsp basil

DIRECTIONS

1. In a bowl combine all ingredients together and mix well
2. In a skillet heat olive oil and pour the egg mixture
3. Cook for 1-2 minutes per side
4. When ready remove omelette from the skillet and serve

Serves: *1*

Prep Time: *5*   Minutes

Cook Time: *10*   Minutes

Total Time: *15*   Minutes

INGREDIENTS

- 2 eggs
- ¼ tsp salt
- ¼ tsp black pepper
- 1 tablespoon olive oil
- ¼ cup cheese
- ¼ tsp basil
- 1 onion

DIRECTIONS

1. In a bowl combine all ingredients together and mix well
2. In a skillet heat olive oil and pour the egg mixture
3. Cook for 1-2 minutes per side
4. When ready remove omelette from the skillet and serve

Serves: *1*

Prep Time: *5* Minutes

Cook Time: *10* Minutes

Total Time: *15* Minutes

INGREDIENTS

- 2 eggs
- ¼ tsp salt
- ¼ tsp black pepper
- 1 tablespoon olive oil
- ¼ cup cheese
- ¼ tsp basil
- 1 cup corn

DIRECTIONS

1. In a bowl combine all ingredients together and mix well
2. In a skillet heat olive oil and pour the egg mixture
3. Cook for 1-2 minutes per side
4. When ready remove omelette from the skillet and serve

Serves: **2**

Prep Time: **5** Minutes

Cook Time: **30** Minutes

Total Time: **35** Minutes

INGREDIENTS

- 1 tsp vanilla extract
- 1 tablespoon honey
- 1 lb. rolled oats
- 2 tablespoons sesame seeds
- ¼ lb. almonds
- ¼ lb. berries

DIRECTIONS

1. Preheat the oven to 325 F
2. Spread the granola onto a baking sheet
3. Bake for 12-15 minutes, remove and mix everything
4. Bake for another 12-15 minutes or until slightly brown
5. When ready remove from the oven and serve

Serves: 2

Prep Time: 5   Minutes

Cook Time: *30*   Minutes

Total Time: *35*   Minutes

INGREDIENTS

- 2 cups oats
- 1 cup almonds
- ¼ cup brown sugar
- 1 tsp cinnamon
- ¼ cup honey
- 1 tsp vanilla essence

DIRECTIONS

1. Preheat the oven to 325 F
2. Spread the granola onto a baking sheet
3. Bake for 12-15 minutes, remove and mix everything
4. Bake for another 12-15 minutes or until slightly brown
5. When ready remove from the oven and serve

Serves: 2

Prep Time: 5 Minutes

Cook Time: 30 Minutes

Total Time: 35 Minutes

INGREDIENTS

- ¼ cup honey
- ½ cup pecans
- 1 cup oats
- 1 tsp vanilla extract
- ¼ cup brown sugar
- 1 tsp orange zest
- ¼ cup cranberries

DIRECTIONS

1. Preheat the oven to 325 F
2. Spread the granola onto a baking sheet
3. Bake for 12-15 minutes, remove and mix everything
4. Bake for another 12-15 minutes or until slightly brown
5. When ready remove from the oven and serve

Serves: 2

Prep Time: 5   Minutes

Cook Time: 30   Minutes

Total Time: 35   Minutes

INGREDIENTS

- 2 cups oats
- ½ cup pumpkin seeds
- ½ cup sesame seeds
- ¼ cup cacao nibs
- ¼ cup coconut flakes
- ¼ cup maple syrup
- 1 cup mixed dried fruits

DIRECTIONS

1. Preheat the oven to 325 F
2. Spread the granola onto a baking sheet
3. Bake for 12-15 minutes, remove and mix everything
4. Bake for another 12-15 minutes or until slightly brown
5. When ready remove from the oven and serve

Serves: **4**

Prep Time: **10** Minutes

Cook Time: **20** Minutes

Total Time: **30** Minutes

INGREDIENTS

- 1 cup whole wheat flour
- ¼ tsp baking soda
- ¼ tsp baking powder
- 2 tablespoons peanut butter
- 2 eggs
- 1 cup milk

DIRECTIONS

1. In a bowl combine all ingredients together and mix well
2. In a skillet heat olive oil
3. Pour ¼ of the batter and cook each pancake for 1-2 minutes per side
4. When ready remove from heat and serve

Serves: **4**

Prep Time: **10**   Minutes

Cook Time: **20**   Minutes

Total Time: **30**   Minutes

INGREDIENTS

- 1 cup whole wheat flour
- ¼ tsp baking soda
- ¼ tsp baking powder
- 1 mashed banana
- 2 eggs
- 1 cup milk

DIRECTIONS

1. In a bowl combine all ingredients together and mix well
2. In a skillet heat olive oil
3. Pour ¼ of the batter and cook each pancake for 1-2 minutes per side
4. When ready remove from heat and serve

Serves: *4*

Prep Time: *10*   Minutes

Cook Time: *20*   Minutes

Total Time: *30*   Minutes

INGREDIENTS

- 1 cup whole wheat flour
- ¼ tsp baking soda
- ¼ tsp baking powder
- 2 eggs
- 1 cup milk

DIRECTIONS

1. In a bowl combine all ingredients together and mix well
2. In a skillet heat olive oil
3. Pour ¼ of the batter and cook each pancake for 1-2 minutes per side
4. When ready remove from heat and serve

Serves: *4*

Prep Time: *10*   Minutes

Cook Time: *20*   Minutes

Total Time: *30*   Minutes

INGREDIENTS

- 1 cup whole wheat flour
- ¼ tsp baking soda
- ¼ tsp baking powder
- ½ mashed mango
- 2 eggs
- 1 cup milk

DIRECTIONS

1. In a bowl combine all ingredients together and mix well
2. In a skillet heat olive oil
3. Pour ¼ of the batter and cook each pancake for 1-2 minutes per side
4. When ready remove from heat and serve

Serves: *1*

Prep Time: *5*   Minutes

Cook Time: *5*   Minutes

Total Time: *10*   Minutes

INGREDIENTS

- ½ cup dried raisins
- ½ cup dried pecans
- ¼ cup almonds
- 1 cup coconut milk
- 1 tsp cinnamon

DIRECTIONS

3. In a bowl combine all ingredients together
4. Serve with milk

Serves: *1*

Prep Time: 5 Minutes

Cook Time: 5 Minutes

Total Time: *10* Minutes

INGREDIENTS

- ½ cup cranberries
- ½ cup dried pecans
- ¼ cup oats
- 1 tablespoon corn cereal
- 1 tsp cinnamon

DIRECTIONS

1. In a bowl combine all ingredients together
2. Serve with milk

Serves: *1*

Prep Time: *5*   Minutes

Cook Time: *5*   Minutes

Total Time: *10*   Minutes

INGREDIENTS

- 1 cup oats
- 1 cup mix dried fruits
- 1 tsp cinnamon
- 1 cup coconut milk

DIRECTIONS

1. In a bowl combine all ingredients together
2. Serve with milk

Serves: *2*

Prep Time: 5   Minutes

Cook Time: *15*   Minutes

Total Time: *20*   Minutes

INGREDIENTS

- ¼ cup egg substitute
- 1 muffin
- 1 turkey sausage patty
- 1 tablespoon cheddar cheese

DIRECTIONS

5. In a skillet pour egg and cook on low heat
6. Place turkey sausage patty in a pan and cook for 4-5 minutes per side
7. On a toasted muffin place the cooked egg, top with a sausage patty and cheddar cheese
8. Serve when ready

Serves: *1*

Prep Time: 5 Minutes

Cook Time: 5 Minutes

Total Time: *10* Minutes

INGREDIENTS

- 2 bread slices
- 6 bacon slices
- 2 fried eggs
- 1 tsp black pepper
- ½ avocado

DIRECTIONS

1. Slightly toast the bread slices
2. Place all the ingredients on a bread slice
3. Top with the other bread slice
4. Toast again until golden brown
5. Serve when ready

Serves: *1*

Prep Time: *5*   Minutes

Cook Time: *5*   Minutes

Total Time: *10*   Minutes

INGREDIENTS

- 2 bread slices
- 2 ham slices
- 1 tablespoon mustard
- 2 fried eggs
- 1 tsp black pepper

DIRECTIONS

1. Slightly toast the bread slices
2. Place all the ingredients on a bread slice
3. Top with the other bread slice
4. Toast again until golden brown
5. Serve when ready

Serves: *1*

Prep Time: *5*   Minutes

Cook Time: *5*   Minutes

Total Time: *10*   Minutes

INGREDIENTS

- 2 bread slices
- 2 tablespoons hummus
- 1 avocado
- 2-3 tomato slices

DIRECTIONS

1. Slightly toast the bread slices
2. Place all the ingredients on a bread slice
3. Top with the other bread slice
4. Toast again until golden brown
5. Serve when ready

Serves: *1*

Prep Time: 5   Minutes

Cook Time: 5   Minutes

Total Time: *10*   Minutes

INGREDIENTS

- 2 bread slices
- 1 carrot
- 1 tablespoon mint
- 2 tablespoons hummus
- 3 tablespoons raisin

DIRECTIONS

1. Slightly toast the bread slices
2. Place all the ingredients on a bread slice
3. Top with the other bread slice
4. Toast again until golden brown
5. Serve when ready

Serves: **8-12**

Prep Time: **10** Minutes

Cook Time: **20** Minutes

Total Time: **30** Minutes

INGREDIENTS

- 2 eggs
- 1 tablespoon olive oil
- 1 cup milk
- 2 cups whole wheat flour
- 1 tsp baking soda
- ¼ tsp baking soda
- 1 tsp cinnamon
- 1 cup strawberries

DIRECTIONS

1. In a bowl combine all dry ingredients
2. In another bowl combine all dry ingredients
3. Combine wet and dry ingredients together
4. Pour mixture into 8-12 prepared muffin cups, fill 2/3 of the cups
5. Bake for 18-20 minutes at 375 F, remove and serve

Serves: *8-12*

Prep Time: *10*   Minutes

Cook Time: *20*   Minutes

Total Time: *30*   Minutes

INGREDIENTS

- 2 eggs
- 1 tablespoon olive oil
- 1 cup milk
- 2 cups whole wheat flour
- 1 tsp baking soda
- ¼ tsp baking soda
- 1 tsp cinnamon
- 1 mashed banana

DIRECTIONS

1. In a bowl combine all dry ingredients
2. In another bowl combine all dry ingredients
3. Combine wet and dry ingredients together
4. Pour mixture into 8-12 prepared muffin cups, fill 2/3 of the cups
5. Bake for 18-20 minutes at 375 F, remove and serve

Serves: **8-12**

Prep Time: **10** Minutes

Cook Time: **20** Minutes

Total Time: **30** Minutes

INGREDIENTS

- 2 eggs
- 1 tablespoon olive oil
- 1 cup milk
- 2 cups whole wheat flour
- 1 tsp baking soda
- ¼ tsp baking soda
- 1 tsp cinnamon
- 1 cup almonds

DIRECTIONS

1. In a bowl combine all dry ingredients
2. In another bowl combine all dry ingredients
3. Combine wet and dry ingredients together
4. Pour mixture into 8-12 prepared muffin cups, fill 2/3 of the cups
5. Bake for 18-20 minutes at 375 F, remove and serve

Serves: *8-12*

Prep Time: *10*   Minutes

Cook Time: *20*   Minutes

Total Time: *30*   Minutes

INGREDIENTS

- 2 eggs
- 1 tablespoon olive oil
- 1 cup milk
- 2 cups whole wheat flour
- 1 tsp baking soda
- ¼ tsp baking soda
- 1 tsp cinnamon
- 1 cup berries

DIRECTIONS

1. In a bowl combine all dry ingredients
2. In another bowl combine all dry ingredients
3. Combine wet and dry ingredients together
4. Pour mixture into 8-12 prepared muffin cups, fill 2/3 of the cups
5. Bake for 18-20 minutes at 375 F, remove and serve

Serves:	**8-12**	
Prep Time:	**10**	Minutes
Cook Time:	**20**	Minutes
Total Time:	**30**	Minutes

INGREDIENTS

- 2 eggs
- 1 tablespoon olive oil
- 1 cup milk
- 2 cups whole wheat flour
- 1 tsp baking soda
- ¼ tsp baking soda
- 1 tsp cinnamon

DIRECTIONS

1. In a bowl combine all dry ingredients
2. In another bowl combine all dry ingredients
3. Combine wet and dry ingredients together
4. Pour mixture into 8-12 prepared muffin cups, fill 2/3 of the cups
5. Bake for 18-20 minutes at 375 F
6. When ready remove from the oven and serve

BREAKFAST COOKIES

Serves: *8-12*

Prep Time: *5*   Minutes

Cook Time: *15*   Minutes

Total Time: *20*   Minutes

INGREDIENTS

- 1 cup rolled oats
- ¼ cup applesauce
- ½ tsp vanilla extract
- 3 tablespoons chocolate chips
- 2 tablespoons dried fruits
- 1 tsp cinnamon

DIRECTIONS

1. Preheat the oven to 325 F
2. In a bowl combine all ingredients together and mix well
3. Scoop cookies using an ice cream scoop
4. Place cookies onto a prepared baking sheet
5. Place in the oven for 12-15 minutes or until the cookies are done
6. When ready remove from the oven and serve

Serves:	*8-12*	
Prep Time:	5	Minutes
Cook Time:	15	Minutes
Total Time:	20	Minutes

INGREDIENTS

- 1 stick butter
- 1 cup brown sugar
- 1 tsp vanilla extract
- 2 eggs
- 2 cups all-purpose flour
- 1 tsp baking soda
- 1 cup chocolate chips

DIRECTIONS

1. Preheat the oven to 325 F
2. In a bowl combine all ingredients together and mix well
3. Scoop cookies using an ice cream scoop
4. Place cookies onto a prepared baking sheet
5. Place in the oven for 12-15 minutes or until the cookies are done
6. When ready remove from the oven and serve

Serves: *8-12*

Prep Time: 5   Minutes

Cook Time: 15   Minutes

Total Time: 20   Minutes

INGREDIENTS

- 1 cup flour
- 1 cup baking soda
- 1 butter stick
- 1 cup brown sugar
- 2 eggs
- 1 cup peanut butter

DIRECTIONS

1. Preheat the oven to 325 F
2. In a bowl combine all ingredients together and mix well
3. Scoop cookies using an ice cream scoop
4. Place cookies onto a prepared baking sheet
5. Place in the oven for 12-15 minutes or until the cookies are done
6. When ready remove from the oven and serve

Serves: *8-12*

Prep Time: *5*   Minutes

Cook Time: *15*   Minutes

Total Time: *20*   Minutes

INGREDIENTS

- 1 cup flour
- ¼ tsp baking powder
- 1 butter stick
- ¼ cup brown sugar
- 1 egg
- 1 tsp vanilla extract
- ½ cup jam

DIRECTIONS

1. Preheat the oven to 325 F
2. In a bowl combine all ingredients together and mix well
3. Scoop cookies using an ice cream scoop
4. Place cookies onto a prepared baking sheet
5. Place in the oven for 12-15 minutes or until the cookies are done
6. When ready remove from the oven and serve

Serves: **8-12**

Prep Time: **5**   Minutes

Cook Time: **15**   Minutes

Total Time: **20**   Minutes

INGREDIENTS

- 1 butter stick
- ½ cup brown sugar
- 1 egg
- 1 tsp vanilla extract
- 1 cup flour
- 1 tsp baking soda
- 1 tsp cinnamon
- 2 cups oats

DIRECTIONS

1. Preheat the oven to 325 F
2. In a bowl combine all ingredients together and mix well
3. Scoop cookies using an ice cream scoop
4. Place cookies onto a prepared baking sheet
5. Place in the oven for 12-15 minutes or until the cookies are done, when ready remove and serve

BANANA BREAKFAST SMOOTHIE

Serves: **1**

Prep Time: **5**   Minutes

Cook Time: **5**   Minutes

Total Time: **10**   Minutes

INGREDIENTS

- ½ cup vanilla yogurt
- 2 tsp honey
- Pinch of cinnamon
- 1 banana
- 1 cup ice

DIRECTIONS

1. In a blender place all ingredients and blend until smooth
2. Pour the smoothie in a glass and serve

Serves: *1*

Prep Time: 5   Minutes

Cook Time: 5   Minutes

Total Time: *10*   Minutes

INGREDIENTS

- ½ cup almonds
- 2 slices peaches
- 1 cup blueberries
- Handful of kale
- 1 cup ice

DIRECTIONS

1. In a blender place all ingredients and blend until smooth
2. Pour the smoothie in a glass and serve

Serves:	*1*
Prep Time:	5 Minutes
Cook Time:	5 Minutes
Total Time:	*10* Minutes

INGREDIENTS

- ½ cup spinach
- 1 cup Greek yogurt
- 1 pear
- ¼ tsp ginger
- 1 cup ice

DIRECTIONS

1. In a blender place all ingredients and blend until smooth
2. Pour the smoothie in a glass and serve

Serves: *1*

Prep Time: 5   Minutes

Cook Time: 5   Minutes

Total Time: *10*   Minutes

INGREDIENTS

- ½ Greek yogurt
- ½ cup oats
- 1 tablespoon pecans
- ¼ tsp nutmeg
- ¼ tsp cinnamon
- 1 apple
- 1 cup ice

DIRECTIONS

1. In a blender place all ingredients and blend until smooth
2. Pour the smoothie in a glass and serve

Serves: *1*

Prep Time: *5*   Minutes

Cook Time: *5*   Minutes

Total Time: *10*   Minutes

INGREDIENTS

- ½ cup yogurt
- 1 tsp honey
- 1 banana
- 1 tsp ginger
- 1 cup ice

DIRECTIONS

1. In a blender place all ingredients and blend until smooth
2. Pour the smoothie in a glass and serve

Serves: *1*

Prep Time: *5* Minutes

Cook Time: *5* Minutes

Total Time: *10* Minutes

INGREDIENTS

- 1 cup vanilla yogurt
- 1 tsp vanilla extract
- 1 orange
- 1 cup ice

DIRECTIONS

1. In a blender place all ingredients and blend until smooth
2. Pour the smoothie in a glass and serve

Serves: *1*

Prep Time: 5   Minutes

Cook Time: 5   Minutes

Total Time: *10*   Minutes

INGREDIENTS

- ¼ cup almond milk
- ¼ cup pitted cherries
- ¼ cup raspberries
- 1 tablespoon honey
- 1 tsp ginger
- 1 cup ice

DIRECTIONS

1. In a blender place all ingredients and blend until smooth
2. Pour the smoothie in a glass and serve

Serves: **1**

Prep Time: 5   Minutes

Cook Time: 5   Minutes

Total Time: **10**   Minutes

INGREDIENTS

- 1 cup vanilla yogurt
- 1 tsp vanilla essence
- 1 cup pineapple juice
- 1 cup pineapple chunks
- 1 cup ice

DIRECTIONS

1. In a blender place all ingredients and blend until smooth
2. Pour the smoothie in a glass and serve

Serves: **1**

Prep Time: 5 Minutes

Cook Time: 5 Minutes

Total Time: **10** Minutes

INGREDIENTS

- 1 cup apple juice
- 1 banana
- 1 kiwi
- 1 strawberry
- 1 cup ice

DIRECTIONS

1. In a blender place all ingredients and blend until smooth
2. Pour the smoothie in a glass and serve

Serves: *1*

Prep Time: 5 Minutes

Cook Time: 5 Minutes

Total Time: *10* Minutes

INGREDIENTS

- 1 cup soy milk
- 1 cup blueberries
- 1 banana
- 1 kiwi
- 1 tsp papaya
- 1 cup ice

DIRECTIONS

1. In a blender place all ingredients and blend until smooth
2. Pour the smoothie in a glass and serve

LYME DISEASE COOKBOOK

40+ Soup, Pizza, and Side Dishes recipes designed for Lyme Disease

SOUP RECIPES

ZUCCHINI SOUP

Serves: **4**

Prep Time: **10** Minutes

Cook Time: **20** Minutes

Total Time: **30** Minutes

INGREDIENTS

- 1 tablespoon olive oil
- 1 lb. zucchini
- ¼ red onion
- ½ cup all-purpose flour
- ¼ tsp pepper
- 1 can vegetable broth
- 1 cup heavy cream

DIRECTIONS

1. In a saucepan heat olive oil and sauté zucchini until tender
2. Add remaining ingredients to the saucepan and bring to a boil
3. When all the vegetables are tender transfer to a blender and blend until smooth
4. Pour soup into bowls, garnish with parsley and serve

Serves: **4**

Prep Time: **10**   Minutes

Cook Time: **20**   Minutes

Total Time: **30**   Minutes

INGREDIENTS

- 1 tablespoon olive oil
- 1 lb. broccoli
- ¼ red onion
- ½ cup all-purpose flour
- ¼ tsp salt
- ¼ tsp pepper
- 1 can vegetable broth
- 1 cup heavy cream

DIRECTIONS

1. In a saucepan heat olive oil and sauté broccoli until tender
2. Add remaining ingredients to the saucepan and bring to a boil
3. When all the vegetables are tender transfer to a blender and blend until smooth
4. Pour soup into bowls, garnish with parsley and serve

Serves: *4*

Prep Time: *10*   Minutes

Cook Time: *20*   Minutes

Total Time: *30*   Minutes

INGREDIENTS

- 1 tablespoon olive oil
- 1 lb. tomato
- ¼ red onion
- ½ cup all-purpose flour
- ¼ tsp salt
- ¼ tsp pepper
- 1 can vegetable broth
- 1 cup heavy cream

DIRECTIONS

1. In a saucepan heat olive oil and sauté tomatoes until tender
2. Add remaining ingredients to the saucepan and bring to a boil
3. When all the vegetables are tender transfer to a blender and blend until smooth
4. Pour soup into bowls, garnish with parsley and serve

Serves: **4**

Prep Time: **10** Minutes

Cook Time: **20** Minutes

Total Time: **30** Minutes

INGREDIENTS

- 1 tablespoon olive oil
- ½ lb. onion
- ¼ red onion
- ½ cup all-purpose flour
- ¼ tsp salt
- 1 lb. carrot
- ¼ tsp pepper
- 1 can vegetable broth
- 1 cup heavy cream

DIRECTIONS

1. In a saucepan heat olive oil and sauté onion until tender
2. Add remaining ingredients to the saucepan and bring to a boil
3. When all the vegetables are tender transfer to a blender and blend until smooth
4. Pour soup into bowls, garnish with parsley and serve

Serves: **4**

Prep Time: **10** Minutes

Cook Time: **20** Minutes

Total Time: **30** Minutes

INGREDIENTS

- 1 tablespoon olive oil
- 1 lb. carrot
- ¼ red onion
- ½ cup all-purpose flour
- ¼ tsp salt
- ¼ tsp pepper
- 1 can vegetable broth
- 1 cup heavy cream

DIRECTIONS

1. In a saucepan heat olive oil and sauté carrots until tender
2. Add remaining ingredients to the saucepan and bring to a boil
3. When all the vegetables are tender transfer to a blender and blend until smooth
4. Pour soup into bowls, garnish with parsley and serve

Serves: *4*

Prep Time: *10*   Minutes

Cook Time: *20*   Minutes

Total Time: *30*   Minutes

INGREDIENTS

- 1 tablespoon olive oil
- 1 lb. cucumber
- ¼ red onion
- ½ cup all-purpose flour
- ¼ tsp salt
- ¼ tsp pepper
- 1 can vegetable broth
- 1 cup heavy cream

DIRECTIONS

1. In a saucepan heat olive oil and sauté cucumber until tender
2. Add remaining ingredients to the saucepan and bring to a boil
3. When all the vegetables are tender transfer to a blender and blend until smooth
4. Pour soup into bowls, garnish with parsley and serve

Serves: *4*

Prep Time: *10*   Minutes

Cook Time: *20*   Minutes

Total Time: *30*   Minutes

INGREDIENTS

- 1 tablespoon olive oil
- 1 lb. shallot
- ¼ red onion
- ½ cup all-purpose flour
- ¼ tsp salt
- ¼ tsp pepper
- 1 can vegetable broth
- 1 cup heavy cream

DIRECTIONS

1. In a saucepan heat olive oil and sauté shallot until tender
2. Add remaining ingredients to the saucepan and bring to a boil
3. When all the vegetables are tender transfer to a blender and blend until smooth
4. Pour soup into bowls, garnish with parsley and serve

Serves: **4**

Prep Time: **10** Minutes

Cook Time: **20** Minutes

Total Time: **30** Minutes

INGREDIENTS

- 1 tablespoon olive oil
- 1 lb. corn
- ¼ red onion
- ½ cup all-purpose flour
- ¼ tsp salt
- ¼ tsp pepper
- 1 can vegetable broth
- 1 cup heavy cream

DIRECTIONS

1. In a saucepan heat olive oil and sauté corn until tender
2. Add remaining ingredients to the saucepan and bring to a boil
3. When all the vegetables are tender transfer to a blender and blend until smooth
4. Pour soup into bowls, garnish with parsley and serve

Serves: **4**

Prep Time: **10** Minutes

Cook Time: **20** Minutes

Total Time: **30** Minutes

INGREDIENTS

- 1 tablespoon olive oil
- 2 lb. red bell pepper
- ¼ red onion
- ½ cup all-purpose flour
- ¼ tsp salt
- ¼ tsp pepper
- 1 can vegetable broth
- 1 cup heavy cream

DIRECTIONS

1. In a saucepan heat olive oil and sauté red bell pepper until tender
2. Add remaining ingredients to the saucepan and bring to a boil
3. When all the vegetables are tender transfer to a blender and blend until smooth
4. Pour soup into bowls, garnish with parsley and serve

GREEN PESTO PASTA

Serves: **2**

Prep Time: **5**   Minutes

Cook Time: **15** Minutes

Total Time: **20** Minutes

INGREDIENTS

- 4 oz. spaghetti
- 2 cups basil leaves
- 2 garlic cloves
- ¼ cup olive oil
- 2 tablespoons parmesan cheese
- ½ tsp black pepper

DIRECTIONS

1. Bring water to a boil and add pasta
2. In a blend add parmesan cheese, basil leaves, garlic and blend
3. Add olive oil, pepper and blend again
4. Pour pesto onto pasta and serve when ready

Serves: 2

Prep Time: 5   Minutes

Cook Time: 15   Minutes

Total Time: 20   Minutes

INGREDIENTS

- 10 oz. spaghetti
- 2 eggs
- ½ cup parmesan cheese
- 1 tsp black pepper
- Olive oil
- 1 tsp parsley
- 2 cloves garlic

DIRECTIONS

1. In a pot boil spaghetti (or any other type of pasta), drain and set aside
2. In a bowl whish eggs with parmesan cheese
3. In a skillet heat olive oil, add garlic and cook for 1-2 minutes
4. Pour egg mixture and mix well
5. Add pasta and stir well
6. When ready garnish with parsley and serve

Serves: **2**

Prep Time: **5**   Minutes

Cook Time: **15**   Minutes

Total Time: **20**   Minutes

INGREDIENTS

- 10 oz. spaghetti
- 2 eggs
- 1 lb. beef
- ½ cup parmesan cheese
- 1 tsp black pepper
- 1 tsp parsley
- 2 cloves garlic

DIRECTIONS

1. In a pot boil spaghetti (or any other type of pasta), drain and set aside
2. In a bowl whish eggs with parmesan cheese
3. In a skillet heat olive oil, add garlic and cook for 1-2 minutes
4. Pour egg mixture and mix well
5. Add pasta, cooked beef and stir well
6. When ready garnish with parsley and serve

Serves: 2

Prep Time: 5   Minutes

Cook Time: 15   Minutes

Total Time: 20   Minutes

INGREDIENTS

- 10 oz. spaghetti
- 2 eggs
- 1 lb. salmon
- ½ cup parmesan cheese
- 1 tsp black pepper
- 1 tsp parsley
- 2 cloves garlic

DIRECTIONS

1. In a pot boil spaghetti (or any other type of pasta), drain and set aside
2. In a bowl whish eggs with parmesan cheese
3. In a skillet heat olive oil, add garlic and cook for 1-2 minutes
4. Pour egg mixture and mix well
5. Add pasta, salmon and stir well
6. When ready garnish with parsley and serve

Serves: 2

Prep Time: 5   Minutes

Cook Time: 15   Minutes

Total Time: 20   Minutes

INGREDIENTS

- 10 oz. spaghetti
- 2 eggs
- 1 lb. cooked chicken breast
- ½ cup parmesan cheese
- 1 tsp black pepper
- 1 tsp parsley
- 2 cloves garlic

DIRECTIONS

1. In a pot boil spaghetti (or any other type of pasta), drain and set aside
2. In a bowl whish eggs with parmesan cheese
3. In a skillet heat olive oil, add garlic and cook for 1-2 minutes
4. Pour egg mixture and mix well
5. Add pasta, cooked chicken breast and stir well
6. When ready garnish with parsley and serve

Serves: *2*

Prep Time: *5*   Minutes

Cook Time: *15*   Minutes

Total Time: *20*   Minutes

INGREDIENTS

- ½ cup celery
- 1 packet Knox Gelatin
- 1 cup cranberry juice
- 1 can berry cranberry sauce
- 1 cup sour cream

DIRECTIONS

1. In a bowl combine all ingredients together and mix well
2. Add dressing and serve

Serves: **2**

Prep Time: **5** Minutes

Cook Time: **15** Minutes

Total Time: **20** Minutes

INGREDIENTS

- 1 tablespoon mustard
- ¼ cup olive oil
- 1 head romaine lettuce
- 2 hard-boiled eggs
- 8 oz. bacon
- 1 avocado
- 6 oz. blue cheese
- 4 oz. tomatoes

DIRECTIONS

1. In a bowl combine all ingredients together and mix well
2. Add dressing and serve

Serves: 2

Prep Time: 5   Minutes

Cook Time: 15   Minutes

Total Time: 20   Minutes

INGREDIENTS

- 1 head cauliflower
- 4 slices bacon
- ¼ cup sour cream
- 1 tablespoon lemon juice
- ¼ tsp garlic powder
- 1 cup cheddar cheese
- 1 tablespoon chopped chives

DIRECTIONS

1. In a bowl combine all ingredients together and mix well
2. Add dressing and serve

Serves: **2**

Prep Time: **5**   Minutes

Cook Time: **15**   Minutes

Total Time: **20**   Minutes

INGREDIENTS

- 1 cup buffalo sauce
- 1 tablespoon honey
- 1 tsp lime
- 1 tsp salt
- 1 tsp onion powder
- 1 tablespoon olive oil
- 1 cup salad dressing

DIRECTIONS

1. In a bowl combine all ingredients together and mix well
2. Add dressing and serve

Serves: *2*

Prep Time: *5*   Minutes

Cook Time: *15*   Minutes

Total Time: *20*   Minutes

INGREDIENTS

- 1 cup farro
- 1 bay leaf
- 1 shallot
- ¼ cup olive oil
- 1 tablespoon apple cider vinegar
- 1 tsp honey
- 1 cup arugula
- 1 apple
- ¼ cup basil
- ¼ cup parsley

DIRECTIONS

1. In a bowl combine all ingredients together and mix well
3. Add dressing and serve

Serves: **2**

Prep Time: **5**   Minutes

Cook Time: **15**   Minutes

Total Time: **20**   Minutes

INGREDIENTS

- 1 lb. carrots
- 1 cup raisins
- ½ cup peanuts
- ½ cup cilantro
- 2 green onions
- ¼ cup olive oil
- 1 tablespoon honey
- 2 cloves garlic
- 1 tsp cumin

DIRECTIONS

1. In a bowl combine all ingredients together and mix well
2. Add dressing and serve

Serves: 2

Prep Time: 5   Minutes

Cook Time: 15   Minutes

Total Time: 20   Minutes

INGREDIENTS

- 1 cup cherry tomatoes
- 1 cucumber
- 1 cup olives
- ¼ red onion
- 1 cup feta
- 1 cup salad dressing

DIRECTIONS

1. In a pan add juice, gelatin, cranberry sauce and cook on low heat
2. Add sour cream, celery and continue to cook
3. Pour mixture into a pan
4. Serve when ready

Serves: *2*

Prep Time: *5*   Minutes

Cook Time: *15*   Minutes

Total Time: *20*   Minutes

INGREDIENTS

- 2 lb. cooked baby potatoes
- 4 slices bacon
- 1 onion
- 1 tablespoon olive oil
- 1 tablespoon mustard
- 1 tsp black pepper

DIRECTIONS

1. In a pan add juice, gelatin, cranberry sauce and cook on low heat
2. Add sour cream, celery and continue to cook
3. Pour mixture into a pan
4. Serve when ready

Serves: 2

Prep Time: 5 Minutes

Cook Time: 15 Minutes

Total Time: 20 Minutes

INGREDIENTS

- 1 avocado
- 1 cup tomatoes
- 1 cucumber
- ½ cup cooked corn
- 1 tablespoon cilantro

DIRECTIONS

1. In a pan add juice, gelatin, cranberry sauce and cook on low heat
2. Add sour cream, celery and continue to cook
3. Pour mixture into a pan
4. Serve when ready

Serves: *1*

Prep Time: *5*   Minutes

Cook Time: *5*   Minutes

Total Time: *10*   Minutes

INGREDIENTS

- 1 cup cottage cheese
- 1 cup sour cream
- 2 green onions
- 2 tsp hot sauce
- 1 tsp dill weed
- ¼ tsp garlic powder
- ½ cup blue cheese

DIRECTIONS

1. In a blender add all ingredients together
2. Blend until smooth
3. Serve when ready

Serves: *1*

Prep Time: 5   Minutes

Cook Time: 5   Minutes

Total Time: *10*   Minutes

INGREDIENTS

- 6 oz. goat cheese
- ½ cup ricotta cheese
- 1 scallion
- 1 tsp lemon zest
- 1 tablespoons lemon juice
- 1 tsp black pepper

DIRECTIONS

1. In a blender add all ingredients together
2. Blend until smooth
3. Serve when ready

Serves: *1*

Prep Time: 5 Minutes

Cook Time: 5 Minutes

Total Time: *10* Minutes

INGREDIENTS

- ½ cup olive oil
- 2 onions
- 3 shallots
- 1 can sour cream
- 1 tablespoon chives
- 1 tsp salt

DIRECTIONS

1. In a blender add all ingredients together
2. Blend until smooth
3. Serve when ready

Serves: *1*

Prep Time: 5   Minutes

Cook Time: 5   Minutes

Total Time: *10*   Minutes

INGREDIENTS

- 2 avocados
- ½ onion
- ½ cup cilantro
- 1 jalapeno
- ½ cup pepitas
- 2 tablespoons lime juice
- 1 tsp salt

DIRECTIONS

1. In a blender add all ingredients together
2. Blend until smooth
3. Serve when ready

Serves: **1**

Prep Time: 5   Minutes

Cook Time: 5   Minutes

Total Time: **10**   Minutes

INGREDIENTS

- 8 oz. cream cheese
- 1 cup Greek yogurt
- ½ cup mayonnaise
- 1 tsp cumin
- 1 tsp paprika
- 1 tsp black pepper
- 1 cup cheddar cheese
- 1 jalapeno pepper

DIRECTIONS

1. In a blender add all ingredients together
2. Blend until smooth
3. Serve when ready

Serves: *1*

Prep Time: 5   Minutes

Cook Time: 5   Minutes

Total Time: *10*   Minutes

INGREDIENTS

- 1 cup sour cream
- ½ cup mayonnaise
- ¼ cup scallions
- 2 tablespoons dill
- 1 tablespoon lemon zest
- 1 tsp black pepper

DIRECTIONS

1. In a blender add all ingredients together
2. Blend until smooth
3. Serve when ready

Serves: *1*

Prep Time: *5*   Minutes

Cook Time: *5*   Minutes

Total Time: *10*   Minutes

INGREDIENTS

- 1 package cream cheese
- 2 tablespoons lemon juice
- 1 tsp salt
- 1 jar pimientos
- 4 oz. Cheddar cheese
- 4 oz. Jack cheese
- 2 scallions
- 1 tsp black pepper

DIRECTIONS

1. In a blender add all ingredients together
2. Blend until smooth
3. Serve when ready

Serves: *1*

Prep Time: *5*   Minutes

Cook Time: *5*   Minutes

Total Time: *10*   Minutes

INGREDIENTS

- 1 cup Greek Yogurt
- 1 tablespoon lemon juice
- 1 tsp black pepper
- 1 scallion
- 1 tablespoon parsley
- 3 oz. blue cheese
- 1 cucumber

DIRECTIONS

1. In a blender add all ingredients together
2. Blend until smooth
3. Serve when ready

ZUCCHINI PIZZA

Serves: **6-8**

Prep Time: **10**   Minutes

Cook Time: **15**   Minutes

Total Time: **25**   Minutes

INGREDIENTS

- 1 pizza crust
- ½ cup tomato sauce
- ¼ black pepper
- 1 cup zucchini slices
- 1 cup mozzarella cheese
- 1 cup olives

DIRECTIONS

1. Spread tomato sauce on the pizza crust
2. Place all the toppings on the pizza crust
3. Bake the pizza at 425 F for 12-15 minutes
4. When ready remove pizza from the oven and serve

Serves: **6-8**

Prep Time: **10** Minutes

Cook Time: **15** Minutes

Total Time: **25** Minutes

INGREDIENTS

- 1 pizza crust
- ½ cup tomato sauce
- ¼ black pepper
- 1 cup salami slices
- 1 cup Brussel sprouts
- 1 cup mozzarella cheese
- 1 cup olives

DIRECTIONS

1. Spread tomato sauce on the pizza crust
2. Place all the toppings on the pizza crust
3. Bake the pizza at 425 F for 12-15 minutes
4. When ready remove pizza from the oven and serve

Serves: *6-8*

Prep Time: *10*   Minutes

Cook Time: *15*   Minutes

Total Time: *25*   Minutes

INGREDIENTS

- 1 pizza crust
- ½ cup tomato sauce
- ¼ black pepper
- 8-9 prosciutto slices
- 1 cup mozzarella cheese
- 1 cup onion

DIRECTIONS

1. Spread tomato sauce on the pizza crust
2. Place all the toppings on the pizza crust
3. Bake the pizza at 425 F for 12-15 minutes
4. When ready remove pizza from the oven and serve

Serves: *6-8*

Prep Time: *10*   Minutes

Cook Time: *15*   Minutes

Total Time: *25*   Minutes

INGREDIENTS

- 1 pizza crust
- ½ cup tomato sauce
- ¼ black pepper
- 1 cup carrot slices
- 1 cup mozzarella cheese
- 1 cup olives

DIRECTIONS

1. Spread tomato sauce on the pizza crust
2. Place all the toppings on the pizza crust
3. Bake the pizza at 425 F for 12-15 minutes
4. When ready remove pizza from the oven and serve

Serves: **6-8**

Prep Time: **10**   Minutes

Cook Time: **15**   Minutes

Total Time: **25**   Minutes

INGREDIENTS

- 1 pizza crust
- ½ cup tomato sauce
- ¼ black pepper
- 1 cup butternut squash
- 1 cup mozzarella cheese
- 1 cup olives

DIRECTIONS

1. Spread tomato sauce on the pizza crust
2. Place all the toppings on the pizza crust
3. Bake the pizza at 425 F for 12-15 minutes
4. When ready remove pizza from the oven and serve

Serves: **6-8**

Prep Time: **10**   Minutes

Cook Time: **15**   Minutes

Total Time: **25**   Minutes

INGREDIENTS

- 1 pizza crust
- ½ cup tomato sauce
- ¼ black pepper
- 3-4 eggs
- 1 cup mozzarella cheese
- 1 cup olives
- 2-3 tomato slices

DIRECTIONS

1. Spread tomato sauce on the pizza crust
2. Place all the toppings on the pizza crust
3. Bake the pizza at 425 F for 12-15 minutes
4. When ready remove pizza from the oven and serve

Serves: **6-8**

Prep Time: **10**   Minutes

Cook Time: **15**   Minutes

Total Time: **25**   Minutes

INGREDIENTS

- 1 pizza crust
- ½ cup tomato sauce
- ¼ black pepper
- 1 cup kale
- 1 cup mozzarella cheese
- 1 cup olives
- 1 cup ricotta

DIRECTIONS

1. Spread tomato sauce on the pizza crust
2. Place all the toppings on the pizza crust
3. Bake the pizza at 425 F for 12-15 minutes
4. When ready remove pizza from the oven and serve

Serves: *6-8*

Prep Time: *10*   Minutes

Cook Time: *15*   Minutes

Total Time: *25*   Minutes

INGREDIENTS

- 1 pizza crust
- ½ cup tomato sauce
- ¼ black pepper
- 1 cup lamb
- 1 cup mozzarella cheese
- 1 cup olives

DIRECTIONS

1. Spread tomato sauce on the pizza crust
2. Place all the toppings on the pizza crust
3. Bake the pizza at 425 F for 12-15 minutes
4. When ready remove pizza from the oven and serve

Serves: *6-8*

Prep Time: *10*   Minutes

Cook Time: *15*   Minutes

Total Time: *25*   Minutes

INGREDIENTS

- 1 pizza crust
- ½ cup tomato sauce
- ¼ black pepper
- 2 anchovy fillets
- 2 garlic cloves
- 1 cup ricotta
- 2 cups kale
- ¼ cup jalapenos
- 1 cup mozzarella cheese
- 1 cup olives

DIRECTIONS

1. Spread tomato sauce on the pizza crust
2. Place all the toppings on the pizza crust
3. Bake the pizza at 425 F for 12-15 minutes
4. When ready remove pizza from the oven and serve

CPSIA information can be obtained
at www.ICGtesting.com
Printed in the USA
BVHW031056050320
574205BV00003B/193